SURVIVORS' GUIDE TO
BREAST CANCER
A COUPLE'S STORY OF FAITH, HOPE, & LOVE

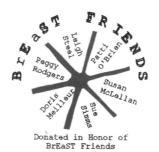

To
Mary and Smitty
Annie Laurie and Dick

Survivors' Guide to Breast Cancer
A Couple's Story of Faith, Hope, & Love

Robert C. Fore, Ed.D
Rorie E. Fore, R.N.

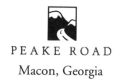

PEAKE ROAD

Macon, Georgia

ISBN 1-57312-170-3
Survivors' Guide to Breast Cancer
A Couple's Story of Faith, Hope, & Love

Robert C. and Rorie E. Fore

Copyright © 1998
Peake Road
Smyth & Helwys Publishing, Inc.
6316 Peake Road
Macon, Georgia 31210-3960
1-800-747-3016

The paper used in this publication meets the minimum
requirements of American Standard for Information Sciences—
Permanence of Paper for Printed Library Material.
ANSI Z39.48–1984.

Library of Congress Cataloging-in-Publication Data
Fore, Robert C.
    Survivors' guide to breast cancer:
    a couple's story of faith, hope, & love/
    Robert C. and Rorie E. Fore.
    p.   cm.
    ISBN 1-57312-170-3 (alk. paper)
    1. Fore, Rorie E.—Health.
    2. Breast—Cancer—Patients—United States—Biography.
    I. Fore, Rorie E.   II. Title.
    RC280.B8F67 1998
    362.1'9699449'0092—dc21
    [B]   97-48563
                                                          CIP

CONTENTS

FOREWORD

Survivors' Guide to Breast Cancer is an awesome story of the role of prayer and faith in healing. For those who have faith, this story reinforces it. For those who are trying to find faith, this account might be a road map. And for those who question the role of faith, this tale might be an opportunity to take another look at their decision. And if the story alone is not enough, the brief allusion to the exciting new research that actually demonstrates the power of prayer, spirituality, and faith is an added reward and reinforcement. This story is timely. One cannot pick up a newspaper or listen to the radio without a reference to the emerging information about spirituality and health.

Many physicians have a rich spiritual life and have quietly included their beliefs in their care patterns over a lifetime of practice. However, the recent research that chronicles the effectiveness of a positive spiritual attitude, of the objective effect of prayer on the morbidity and mortality of patients, is literature that many may not have read or may have discounted. It is a literature that ought to accompany stories such as this lest a reader discount the message as speculation or a missed diagnosis.

For example, a 1996 Duke University study concluded that older people who attend religious services are less likely to be depressed and are physically healthier. In 1988, Randolph Byrd at San Francisco General Medicine Center Hospital reported a study involving 393 coronary care patients who were randomly assigned to either a prayer intervention group or a control group. Those in the "prayed for" group were recipients of prayer from Protestants and Catholics who did not know and were not known by the patients. This study, reported in the *Southern Medical Journal*, showed that the daily prayer group had fewer complications and life-threatening events than the control group. Furthermore, the "prayed for" patients had fewer cardiac arrests, less congestive heart failure, and fewer cases of pneumonia.

In the mid-1990s, the Templeton Foundation awarded "faith and medicine" grants to five medical schools, including the prestigious Johns Hopkins Medical School, to support teaching on health care and spirituality. Up to one fourth of the nation's medical schools now offer courses that address spirituality. Perhaps this is a start to both enhancing the humanity of health care providers and quantifying or objectifying the premise set forth by Rorie and Robert Fore.

One of the most important messages of the Fores' book is the strong, repeated reminder that denial and delay can be deadly. Rorie was lucky . . . she was blessed that her denial did not cost her life. Her courage in speaking out may save other lives. But ultimately, each of us must realize that our fears may cause us to avoid the very intervention that could save us. Rorie's admonition cannot be repeated often enough. Cancer *can* happen to you and to me. We can intellectually understand the importance of seeking medical intervention and still emotionally lie to ourselves and hide from knowledge. Even as we vow to protect ourselves, we also must reach out a firm hand to our friends, family members, and neighbors to bolster their choice not to delay or deny. Sharing this message in an easy-to-read "people next door" story might carry home the moral.

For members of the health care industry, this book is a poignant tale that communicates the immense importance of the relationships and attitudes we carry into patient rooms. How very often Rorie was uplifted by a smile, an encouraging word, or a pat on the shoulder by someone on her care team. And how long she remembered the rare instance of thoughtlessness or careless comment. While physicians, nurses, therapists, and others spend long years learning the science of our professions, we must not forget that the humanity we bring to the science is as powerful a tool as chemotherapy or scalpel. In this day and time of bottom lines threatening physician decision making and disembodied voices making judgments about treatments and interventions, this story is a quiet reminder that humanity and caring cost little and add nothing to the bill. Why, we haven't even found a billing code for encouragement and compassion!

As an officer of the American Medical Association, I am encouraged by the remarkable tale of the professionalism, compassion, and competence shown by the members of the profession of medicine portrayed in this story. As our society struggles with managed care, access to care, and cost of care, it is refreshing to find a portrayal of our profession that I believe is the norm and not an oddity. However, in a day when every physician is being pressed to move faster, see more patients, and spend less time, *Survivors' Guide to Breast Cancer* might serve as a measuring stick of whether or not we are keeping our priorities in order. Are we making sure that meeting the needs of the patient comes first? Are we taking the time (unreimbursable) to answer that lingering question or to provide the extra reassurance? Are we encouraging patients to have preventive care and appropriate follow-up done even if the incentives are to do less? In this day of rapid change in the health care delivery system, it is imperative that the strong foundation of medical ethics and professionalism remain the cornerstone of medicine.

Survivors' Guide to Breast Cancer is a must read.

- For men and women, it reminds us that fear is a bigger enemy than cancer.
- For women, it reminds us that the beauty of the person comes from within, even as the threat of loss of femininity and sexuality seems more pronounced.
- For men, it provides a model of support, understanding, and adoration.
- For physicians and nurses, it provides the humanity that enriches the science.
- For those who question the presence of a greater power, it points to a force with which to be reckoned.

Nancy W. Dickey, M.D.
President-Elect
American Medical Association

PREFACE

One becomes an expert out of desire or necessity. After months of denial, we became reluctant experts on breast cancer. We learned that breast cancer is the second leading cause of cancer death for all women and the leading cause of cancer death for women between the ages of 40 and 55. In the United States alone, 1 out of 8 women will develop breast cancer, and it is newly diagnosed every 3 minutes. A woman dies from breast cancer every 12 minutes.

As two professionals in the health care arena, we should have been more informed and more sensitive to the symptoms of this devastating disease. But we were like many couples who are seduced into believing that nothing is wrong. Breast cancer happens to other people, not us.

In many ways our story is typical, and in many ways it is extraordinary. When the diagnosis was confirmed, we were fortunate to be surrounded by a health care system driven by doctors and nurses who were our friends. We knew who to seek, and we knew how to take charge of the complicated array of treatment options and services. We had adequate health insurance and even had a cancer policy that went into effect just prior to the diagnosis.

The progression from symptoms to diagnosis to treatment is experienced by thousands of women. But as we journeyed through each stage of treatment toward recovery, it became clear that God was moving in our lives, and we had a story to tell that might offer encouragement to couples struggling through the same circumstance. Our story is not just about a husband and wife who found themselves in a predicament that was unlike any crisis they had ever faced. This story is about hundreds of caring people who hate breast cancer and love those who fight it. We have named many of them throughout. Perhaps even more who shared our grief and joy are not mentioned by name, but they will reside forever in our hearts. This is a story about breast cancer. And it is a story about faith and hope. But most of all, it is a story about love.

—Robert and Rorie Fore

There are three things that last forever:
faith, hope, and love;
and the greatest of these is love.
(1 Cor 13:13 REV)

SYMPTOMS
Recognizing the Enemy

"There is in every true woman's heart a spark of heavenly fire, which lies dormant in the broad daylight of prosperity; but which kindles up, and beams and blazes in the dark hour of adversity."

—Washington Irving

This is very difficult. I wish I could be planning another trip to Greece where I lived as an Army brat or simply working every day as a nurse where I could enjoy my patients and go home to a glass of wine and my wonderful family. But in the last year or so, life has not been so generous.

As long as I can remember, I have detected lumps in my breasts. Robert and I were newlyweds in Jacksonville, Florida, twenty-six years ago when my gynecologist informed me that I had fibrocystic disease. My right breast always seemed to be the problem, being the most sensitive before each menstrual period. Even as an adolescent, the doctor said the noticeable lump in my right breast was just the result of my rapidly changing body.

The years passed. I followed my philosophy of looking for fun in everything life had to offer. If a good time wasn't part of the agenda, I wasn't interested. On rare but unmistakable occasions, a dark cloud of worry would pass over me concerning breast trouble, but I managed to overcome any temptation to panic, moving quickly on to whatever seemed to offer the most promise for fun.

In 1970, Robert and I were married. We were blessed with our son Brooke in 1972, and with Jessica in 1979. We started out in Jacksonville and then moved to Athens, Georgia, where Robert completed his doctorate and we embraced the ritual of Georgia "Bulldawg" football. Then we returned home to Jacksonville. Later we moved to Macon, Georgia, then back to Jacksonville, and five years later, back to Macon. We've had an exceptional marriage, and we've been enveloped in happiness.

Before I married, I lived at home with my parents in Jacksonville and could look out my bedroom window and see the house next door and two more across the street as the road curved around under huge oak trees. I mention those houses because in each house lived and died a woman with breast cancer. My father died of multiple myeloma in 1982. A bit further around the circle lived a couple who were our good friends. She died of breast cancer, and he died of prostate cancer. Robert is convinced that my little corner of the neighborhood must be built on top of some kind of toxic waste. I can't help but wonder if my years at home exposed me to something that has placed me in this predicament.

I never talked about it, but I was deeply affected by the fact that all those women seemed to be diagnosed early, treated aggressively, and died almost as though on schedule two or three years later. What hurt the most was my next door neighbor, Anne Lynn, who in her late forties found a lump, had an immediate mastectomy, then chemotherapy, and was gone in two years. She was very pretty, highly educated, and had an unforgettable wit and charm. She never smoked and lived a happy, healthy life. How could this happen? I was profoundly affected, and I absorbed a lethal dose of fear that I have carried with me since.

I always wanted to be a nurse. I could have pursued that objective when I graduated from Robert E. Lee High School, but I went to junior college and, well, let's just say my fun-loving philosophy cut my college career short. I went to work at a bank, and soon I was married. Brooke was born two years later. When he kept coming home from the daycare center with all kinds of bugs, I decided to become a full-time mother. That is a decision I maintained through Jessica's birth and childhood and one I have never regretted. Living on one paycheck all those years was extremely difficult, but we always had everything we needed.

In 1989, Robert was advancing professionally and encouraged me to fulfill my dream and become a nurse. The kids were much older, and I could get student loans from the state of Georgia and the Medical Center where Robert worked. If I eventually went to work at the Medical Center, I could have all my loans forgiven through service. What an opportunity, I thought, so I eagerly entered nursing school. The fun-loving kid who never went to class had finally grown up. I even made the dean's list. I couldn't get enough of school. I loved every minute. I was very happy, and my family did all they could to support and help me. I graduated in 1992, bought myself a hot little sports car, and went to work in Outpatient Surgery. I had everything I wanted. Life looked better than ever.

About a year before graduation, I went for a regular checkup and Pap smear. My gynecologist suggested a mammogram due to a questionable area in my right breast. He thought it wasn't malignant, and the mammogram proved him right. But he wanted an ultrasound, anyway. The x-rays showed multiple cysts that looked like clumps of grapes. The radiologist shook his head, smiled, and said I had absolutely nothing to worry about. Thanks, Doc, I'm out of here! A year later I had another mammogram and ultrasound. Still no problem, I was told, but the grapes had become more numerous. Again, I went home relieved and reassured.

I walked into the Medical Center as a new registered nurse in August 1992, a bit nervous and unsure, but ready to work hard and learn everything I could to be successful. In a very short time I felt confident and comfortable in my new environment. I loved going to work every day. I met so many interesting people with fascinating stories to tell. I felt energized. My days were full with work and my responsibilities to my family at home. Because of my schedule, I had a convenient excuse to postpone regular checkups and always promised to go next month. Several times I actually made an appointment just to make Robert happy, but some kind of real or imagined conflict would always come up at the last minute, and I would cancel.

My troublesome right breast became more firm and tender as if to remind me it was not going to leave me alone. Even though I see cancer every day, I tapped into whatever lingering denial I had left and convinced myself that the "grapes" were nothing. Robert and I would get into arguments about my delaying tactics, and finally I couldn't postpone a doctor's appointment any longer.

In May 1995, I decided to see Dr. Teresa Luhrs, a new obstetrician-gynecologist who had completed her residency at the Medical Center. I had never had a female doctor, but I liked the idea. I was not surprised when she told me I had a firmness in my right breast and should schedule a mammogram. But I did not go. I will never know if those grapelike lumps had already turned into cancer invading my normal breast cells on the way to my lymph nodes. And if I had breast cancer then, I'll never know if I could have had a lumpectomy alone.

Why didn't I make that appointment? Maybe my mind took me back to Jacksonville, and I looked out my bedroom window and saw

Anne Lynn in her backyard playing with her two daughters. Maybe I thought that once a doctor says cancer, the schedule is set, and a two-year limit on life begins. A reservoir of fear can play tricks on the mind, and someone who should know better can think of a thousand reasons to avoid doing what has to be done. After all, we had a vacation planned at Panama City Beach over the 4th of July. Brooke's precious girlfriend, Leah, would be going with us. We would have a memorable holiday. Then it would be time for football season—and we just don't miss Georgia football games, not when my husband is referred to as "Dr. Dawg." Then Christmas would be here, and after that I would be going with Jessica on a school trip to Greece. I could not and would not let the possibility of cancer and all that horrible disease brings with it interfere with my life. At once I began to savor every moment of those experiences while I was consumed by a terrible sense of dread.

One night I came to bed and started crying as I lay there in Robert's arms. That's not something I often do. I cry at weddings and over sad movies, but I can usually control my emotions when it comes to my own troubles. Robert thought I had had an unusually bad day at work, but I didn't tell him that the dread and fear I was carrying around had caught up with me.

Every morning when I walked down the driveway to get the newspaper at 5:00 A.M., I would pray to God not to let the growing lump in my right breast be cancer. Then I would feel better and get through the day. Then several months later, I began having a clear discharge from my right nipple that became more profuse over succeeding weeks. I also noticed a small crease over the top of the right side of my breast that itched, and the skin was flushed. As a nurse, I had lots of information on breast cancer, so I conveniently diagnosed myself as having a nonmalignant condition. I eagerly dismissed what were classic symptoms of breast cancer.

Robert had finally had enough. He had been patient much too long. He insisted that I go to the doctor. No excuses, no procrastination, he was going to call my doctor himself if I didn't. He was angry because he was afraid, and I broke down and cried again. Robert assured me that he understood I was scared, but the time had come. I called the Regional Imaging Center and made an appointment. This time my husband would go with me.

Several weeks before, we decided to go to a Johnny Mathis concert in Atlanta at Chastain Park. It was on a Wednesday evening. We planned to leave work early. We had never been to Chastain Park, so we studied the directions carefully so we wouldn't get lost. We packed wine and little corned beef and turkey sandwiches and took a red candle to light on our folding Bulldawg table when the sun went down. Of course, we got lost. And like most men, Robert wouldn't ask for directions, so we put an extra twenty miles on my Camaro trying to find the concert. We somehow arrived on time. Johnny Mathis sang all the old songs we loved when we were dating and then as newlyweds. Near the end of the show, Robert said he felt faint, and his heartbeat was racing. He had a frightening anxiety attack and was almost ready to go see one of the medics posted near the crowd. He wanted to go home. To our relief, he felt much better when we got back to the car. I knew he was terrified about my mammogram the next day.

I will always think of June 6, 1996, as the beginning of our story. I was a wreck when Robert and I arrived for my mammogram. The radiology technician was very kind, and she knew immediately that I had a serious problem. She was gentle, thank goodness, and didn't hurt me at all. I was focused on my right breast and was devastated when she said they needed some extra films of my *left* breast. This lady was a stranger, but I told her about my fears and that I knew I would need to have a biopsy. I left with a welcome feeling of relief. I was actually going to do something about this awful distraction in my life. I was tired of my denial and wanted to move forward.

Jessica had plans to go on a church choir tour. The group's first stop would be Panama City Beach. Robert and I hadn't been on a vacation alone in years, so several weeks prior to Jessica's trip, we decided we would drive down to Panama City Beach, too. We would be alone, and Jessica would be with her church group in another motel about a mile away. We tried to enjoy every minute, but I felt as if a heavy hour glass was on a chain around my neck as we got closer to going home.

The night before we left, Robert and I were sitting on the beach waiting for the sunset. Out of nowhere a man walked up and asked if we would like for him to take our picture. The photograph he took has become one of my most valuable possessions. In it we're sitting close together surrounded by beautiful sunlight. Our feet are buried in sparkling sand. My dark brown hair is long and full. We look like a couple on their honeymoon. Maybe that man who came out of nowhere was an angel who knew we needed to hold on to that special moment. I'll never forget that weekend as long as I live. It was wonderful, but it had an uneasy finality about it because I knew our lives would never be the same.

From Robert . . .

I think the first time I saw Rorie Smith was when I was eighteen years old and working in a clothing store while attending junior college. This attractive high school senior would come in, and I was always taken by her smile. She was always smiling and had an intangible quality about her that stirred my interest. Who was this girl who was so happy and self-assured? I was very much involved with another girl at the time, so Rorie Smith was just someone I looked for and enjoyed seeing in the store, but I didn't think she even knew my name.

It wasn't long before the girl I had loved for three years proved that she didn't love me, and, as so often in youth, the marriage that was to be never happened. I eventually graduated from the University of South Florida in Tampa and came back home to Jacksonville as a special education teacher. Since my teaching salary in 1969 was a whopping $6,000 a year, I went back to work at night and on weekends in the same clothing store. I was still licking my wounds over my broken engagement and was very lonely.

I will never forget the night that Rorie Smith reappeared and walked a few steps into the store wearing shorts and a paint-covered T-shirt. To my great delight, she seemed to recognize me. She invited me to walk down the mall to look at a Volkswagen she was painting for an art class project at the local junior college. The smile was still there. In a week or two I called her. She already had a date but asked me to call again, which I did. Our first date was Thanksgiving weekend, 1969. We went to a drive-in movie to see *Change of Habit* with Elvis Presley and Mary Tyler Moore. Several of my fraternity brothers were in town, and they followed us in a gigantic old Jeep and then sat on the ground under blankets right next to my car. This was a most impressive scene for a first date.

Rorie's father, who would eventually become the best friend I ever had, didn't like me. He told Rorie not to have anything to do with "that fellow." Her mother was at best cautiously optimistic. At that time in my life I was a bit shy and lacked some self-confidence, which came across as conceit and self-centeredness. I was also still feeling sorry for myself because I had been bitterly hurt. I imagine I was just a tad too perfect with my light blue button-down shirt, khaki pants, and weejuns. I bought a new 1969 Pontiac Firebird with an 8-track tape player and some flashy new clothes. I was going to be a real man about town.

Rorie Smith wanted to have fun. And with all my imperfections, she loved me. Before long, I knew I loved her, too. I have learned to believe in guardian angels, and I believe there was an angel in the mall that night who whispered to Rorie to walk by the clothing store and check out the sale. If she hadn't been there that night painting flowers on a Volkswagen, we probably would have never crossed paths. Rorie's walking into that store that night was one of the defining moments of my life.

On August 8, 1970, I found myself thumbing through a copy of the *Methodist Hymnal* looking for the service of holy matrimony. Though I knew it was a simple service and the minister would tell me exactly what to say, I wanted to be well-rehearsed. In an hour or so I would put on a new suit and drive to Ortega United Methodist Church where my life would change forever. I was excited and scared. I wanted to be a good husband ready for on-the-job training.

I stood up in front of God, my parents, Rorie's parents, the Reverend Rudolph McKinley, and a fair-sized crowd and made the biggest promise of my life. In front of everybody, I promised "to have and to hold, from this day forward, for better or worse, for richer, for poorer, in sickness and in health, to love and to cherish" until we are parted by death. That was a tall order for a twenty-two-year-old kid. But I am absolutely sure I have become a much better human being because of my life with Rorie.

It has never been her nature to criticize, even though I have made some terrible decisions during our marriage. When I've felt defeated, she has always given me courage. Rorie has a remarkable ability to be happy and make everyone around her feel good. And most of all, she has an unwavering faith in God.

Early in our marriage we moved at least once a year. Our joke was that when it was time for a new pizza pan, it was time to move. I kept going to school at night and in the summer and eventually earned a master of education degree from the University of Florida, and then was awarded a doctoral fellowship to the University of Georgia. I quit my job, and Rorie, eighteen-month-old Brooke and I headed to Athens where we moved into married housing. This was truly a unique phase of our lives. Somehow we lived on just more than $450 a month. Our main diet consisted of pizza, Krystal burgers, and beer.

About midway into the 1973 football season, we discovered that it was a source of great entertainment to walk the half mile or so to Sanford Stadium and watch the Georgia Bulldawgs, then come home and cook out. No matter what we cooked out, about midnight it would be time for some Krystal burgers with our upstairs neighbors, Claudia and Rusty Shearer.

Those days resulted in our lifelong love for the Bulldawgs. We cultivated close friendships over the years as we tailgated at each home game with people we would have never met otherwise. Football is a way of life in the Southeastern Conference, and people make important life decisions around the schedule of their favorite team. We love all that surrounds football season because it is far more than the games themselves. Georgia football is tailor-made for someone who enjoys life as much as Rorie. Now Jessica has headed to Athens, working toward a journalism degree and a career in front of a camera or on stage.

So we've certainly had the better and worse, some of the richer and lots of the poorer, the health, and finally we encountered the sickness part. When people marry, they're caught up in romance and optimism, and the future looks as though they will live happily ever after. I think far too few couples really think about what they're promising when they stand at the altar. Trouble has a way of raising its ugly head when you least expect it.

Our marriage has been blessed in many ways. Some might even say we've been lucky. People have actually told me they think Rorie and I are the perfect couple. There's no such thing. We've had plenty of hurdles to jump. Although our main problem has been financial, we've managed to overcome that in the last few years since Rorie graduated from nursing school and added an extra paycheck. Rorie has been a wonderful mother, and together we've raised two children who are successful and have integrity. Though we've had problems like everyone else, life has been good. But suddenly we found ourselves facing the challenge of our lives.

Sometimes anger and fear can be confused because they both take a toll and can feel the same. I was afraid that Rorie had cancer, and I was angry that she avoided a mammogram while a lump in her breast grew larger and larger. This didn't happen overnight. I remember that in September or October 1995, Rorie's usual lumpy right breast began to change. It was a noticeable change that created a visible and distinct crease in her breast.

I begged her to have it checked, and she promised she would after Christmas. That was such a typical response from a girl who had always lived for the moment and had an unlimited capacity to postpone the unpleasant. Rorie's love for the moment was one of the things I found so attractive about her. But I felt like we were in trouble, and it was no time to stop and smell the roses.

Christmas came and went. Her breast became more distorted along with the beginning of a small ulceration. My pleas for her to see a doctor were answered with "right after Jessica and I return from Greece." They had an exciting trip, but Rorie's breast got worse.

Our lovemaking wasn't affected, except that she was becoming more and more self-conscious and would try to keep her breast covered with her nightgown. The only time she would remove her nightgown was when the lights were off. After twenty-five years of marriage, Rorie suddenly didn't want me to see her in the bathtub or shower.

My frustration grew as I couldn't understand how a registered nurse who saw cancer every day could avoid what had to be done. There I was, a director of medical education in a major teaching hospital, and I was helpless. I knew we were in big trouble, but Rorie just would not go to the doctor. I tried everything in my arsenal from the silent treatment to threats, but nothing worked. Her avoidance and denial convinced me even more that she knew this was very serious. She could no longer make light of how she always had lumpy breasts and assure me that she had a little problem with fibrocystic disease. The time had come for the inevitable. I knew it was a virtual certainty: my wife had breast cancer. But in all those months of worrying and arguing, I never used the word "cancer." It was as though if I said it, it would come true.

I saw Dr. Luhrs one evening just by chance while I was attending a dinner meeting. She was with her husband, and I hesitated to interrupt her. But I asked if I could speak to her privately. I told her about my concerns and fears. She promised she would call Rorie and see if she could find out what was going on. I was so relieved with Dr. Luhrs' calm, confident approach. I knew that soon the postponing would be over. Rorie had to make the decision, and finally she did.

We made an appointment for a mammogram. Rorie and I agreed that Thursday, June 6, 1996, marked a new beginning in our life together. Our first twenty-six years came to a close two months later, and we have memory after memory to cherish. Music always brings back memories. Several weeks before, we made plans to attend a Johnny Mathis concert in Atlanta. We remember him way back in the early sixties with "Chances Are," "Wonderful, Wonderful," and "The Twelfth of Never." This was going to be a big night out, and we carefully planned everything well in advance. We were particularly concerned about not getting lost on the way to Chastain Park. Rorie will claim that we did, but I prefer to report that we were temporarily directionally challenged. Anyway, we arrived on time, and the concert was all we expected.

To my great disappointment and frustration, however, I could never relax and enjoy the music. As the last hour of the concert approached, I began to have the worst anxiety attack of my life. My pulse raced, and I found it difficult to breathe. I was at such a stage of panic that I was ready to go to the medic tent, but I simultaneously wanted to avoid ending up in an Atlanta hospital and not being able to return home. Rorie was terribly concerned, but I don't think she ever realized how much that episode frightened me. I don't think I had a heart attack because I didn't have chest pain, but a heart attack couldn't have been worse. I was so concerned about Rorie that my fear became overwhelming. I'm thankful that we got back home and I felt much better. But I didn't sleep at all thinking about the next day.

I am sure Rorie was trying her best to hide her fear as we drove into the Regional Imaging Center parking lot. As we got out of the car and walked toward the entrance, we nervously laughed about how we felt like school kids being sent to the principal's office. Laughter and humor have always been a mainstay of our marriage, and that day we needed it. We checked in at the desk, and Rorie was ushered back into the examination area almost immediately. I sat alone and thumbed through some magazines, unable to think of anything else but what might lie ahead. I kept repeating in the back of my mind, "Maybe the lump isn't malignant; maybe it's not malignant." But I knew better. With all our worry about Rorie's right breast, the mammography session resulted in extra films of her left breast. Our fears were multiplying. The truth was closing in.

I wanted to take Rorie and escape to the beach for the weekend before the final mammography report arrived. We needed to be alone. How many years had it been since we were able to go to the beach by ourselves? Our vacations had always been family affairs including Rorie's mother and father until he died. Rorie loves the beach, and we kind of made an unspoken pact that weekend to live every minute to its fullest. The first day was quite cloudy and dreary, but we were determined to have fun. We didn't speak about the report waiting for us, and we held hands and touched more than usual. I think Rorie was terrified, and I was numb. But the sunset our last night was spectacular. We took picture after picture as the sun seemed to be slowly devoured by the gulf. It was as though we knew we would never look at another sunset quite the same again. Everything we would see and feel from that day on would be in the context of cancer . . . fearing it, fighting it, and remembering it.

DIAGNOSIS
Facing the Truth

"We could never learn to be brave and patient, if there were only joy in the world."

—Helen Keller

From Rorie . . .

The long uneventful drive back to Macon from Panama City gets us home late Monday afternoon. Robert and I have barely unpacked when the telephone rings. Our hearts pound as I listen to Dr. Luhrs, who sounds almost out of breath. I can tell from her voice that the report in front of her is forcing her to make a call she wishes had never been necessary. "Highly suspicious for cancer in right breast, questionable area in left breast." I hear the words I have expected for so long, but I still am not prepared. I cry, and Robert is fighting tears as he wraps his arms around me. In a moment or two we begin to collect our thoughts and start reaching for the courage we will need for many months to come.

All the avoidance and denial are finally over. Now it begins, I think. My prayers are apparently being answered because my coping skills allow me to instantly remove part of myself from the situation and start viewing events as much as a spectator as the central character. I am quickly developing the ability to step back when faced with painful information and draw into my deepest being where I encounter a connection with Jesus stronger than I could have ever imagined. Of course, I can still feel pain and anguish, but it isn't as debilitating as I prepared for it to be.

The first images racing through my mind are how much I dread telling Brooke and Jessica and seeing their reactions. And I can't stand the idea of calling my mother, Mary, in Jacksonville. Her mother died of ovarian cancer, and my father died of multiple myeloma. Now I am going to have to tell her that her daughter has breast cancer. Brooke will be home in a few hours, and Jessica is still on her church choir tour. If she calls, and surely she will as she does every day, I won't tell her over the telephone. I have to tell her in person, and I will do it as soon as she walks in the door. When Brooke finally comes home, I tell him. He seems to accept the news in a way to reassure me. I feel better knowing that I am beginning the process of telling my family and friends.

I go to work Tuesday morning as if all is well. I have an appointment for 9:00 A.M. Wednesday morning with Dr. Paul Dale, a young surgeon who specializes in surgical oncology. I get through the day and act as if nothing is bothering me. In many ways, very little is bothering me. Over the previous few weeks I prayed constantly and asked Jesus to give me strength and help me to be calm as the dreadful news starts to pile up. I want to be strong for myself and my family, and I need Jesus to be with me so this awful disease won't defeat me. I am convinced my prayers are being answered because I begin to feel Jesus with me as if he has his hand gently on my shoulder. I feel a sense of peace.

Robert and I walk into Dr. Dale's office at precisely 9:00 A.M. His office is located in the Doctors Building adjacent to the Surgery Center where I work. His office manager, Sharon, is positive and cheerful, and we become instant friends. She wants to talk, and so do I. Not all doctors appreciate how important their front office staff is in helping patients feel as relaxed and comfortable as possible. I talk to front office staff in doctor's offices almost every day, and some act as though it's a chore to answer a simple question. Unfortunately, some doctors don't seem to be aware of how much they are helped or hurt by the person who answers the telephone.

In a few minutes we are ushered into an examining room. I change into a gown while Robert tries to act confident with his little pats on my knee and a smile. I can hear Dr. Dale arrive as he checks with Sharon on some details, and then he opens the door as I say another instant prayer. I like this young man's bedside manner. He immediately puts me at ease. But I feel terribly self-conscious as he examines my breasts. First, he asks me to lower my gown. He carefully looks at me as I sit up on the examining table. I am bracing myself for a lecture about how I waited too long and I should have seen a doctor sooner and what about the ulcer on my breast and on and on. But this doctor is sensitive enough to know that he doesn't have to say anything. All he wants me to know is that he is going to use all his knowledge and skills to help me.

I wonder how Robert feels as I sit there naked from the waist up going through a breast examination. He has never been with me during a physical examination, but I sense he will be with me for every doctor's appointment from now on. I know this is difficult for him.

Then I have to lie on my back as Dr. Dale feels for lumps in each breast. The lump in my right breast and the ulcer are obvious indicators of trouble. The lump in the left breast, if any, is not so evident. After a thorough exam, Dr. Dale asks us to follow him to view the results of my mammogram. He gently explains what we are looking at and gives us a short but understandable lesson on how to read the films. Then we return to the examining room.

Dr. Dale's voice is soft and steady as he looks at me and says he is sure I have cancer in the right breast, and a biopsy will be necessary to determine any cancer in the left breast. He nods slowly as he talks in a manner to assure me he will get me through all this. The biopsy will be on Monday, and there may be a possibility of a bilateral mastectomy on Wednesday. Once again, I know my many prayers are answered because I am calm as I listen and remember all he says. My first words are questions about breast reconstruction. Dr. Dale arranges for me to see a plastic and reconstructive surgeon, Dr. Roy Powell, at 4:00 P.M. this afternoon.

As Robert and I leave the office and walk into the hallway, we awkwardly try to reassure each other that everything will be fine. He squeezes my hand as we decide to go back to work for a while. I return to Outpatient Holding on the second floor of the Surgery Center. My nurse friends and co-workers are anxiously waiting on the verdict. These women have become my dear friends. The Medical Center is addressing diversity issues among its workforce. I suppose it's a good idea across the organization. Many of my co-workers are black, and we laugh about our racial and cultural differences and similarities. What matters on this day is the fact that we are all women. The tears we shed together when I tell them the results prove that we share a common bond and we love each other. They will never know how much I need them and how they comfort me.

Robert and I eat lunch together as we do most every day. It is wonderful being able to work in the same place so we can eat lunch together and see each other during the day. The news about me is already spreading through the Surgery Center. I see co-workers in the cafeteria who have breast cancer. There are so many. What is going on? Hardly a week goes by that we don't hear about someone else being diagnosed. What's causing all this? Is there a pattern? I don't know. I look around and wonder who knows about me and who doesn't.

The day drags on and on. Finally it is time to leave to see Dr. Powell. I know him from my work in the Surgery Center and have seen the results of his breast reconstruction skills on many of my patients. Also, he is a member of our church. His office is located in a medical complex near where we live, so we take the route we always take to go home. When we arrive, we wait a few minutes and then are taken back into a small room that is used for patient education. We watch a videotape on breast reconstruction and talk briefly to a nurse who asks me some questions about my medical history. Is this day ever going to end? I am getting weary, and I know Robert is getting by on nerves alone.

We are then taken to the second examination room of the day. I go through the now familiar routine of taking off my blouse and bra and putting on a robe. Robert will once again have to sit close by while my breasts are probed and measured. He tries to joke that he wonders if by the end of the day there will be anyone left in Macon who hasn't seen my breasts. Probably not, I think, probably not.

Roy comes in and appears to be shocked that this is me sitting in his examination room. He shakes Robert's hand and holds my hand as he expresses his sincerest regrets that breast cancer has brought us to him. I say another prayer, thanking God that if I have to be in this predicament, how blessed I am to have a member of my church as one of my doctors. Roy is very concerned about me, but his professional demeanor takes over as he knows there are many questions and many options. The mass in my right breast appears to be quite large, about 5 cm. He thinks that reconstruction may have to be delayed because of the probability of chemotherapy and even radiation. I am very demoralized because I have planned for everything to work out perfectly. I will have a double mastectomy and reconstruction all in the same day, and in a few weeks I will be ready to show off my new, better-than-ever body. Heck, I might even get a tummy tuck wrapped up in the deal and look ten years younger. But the facts are causing my lofty plans to crash down to earth. Robert and I leave exhausted and discouraged as the reality of our situation is starting to take a toll.

I realize this will not be just an inconvenience that lasts only a few weeks. I am facing a very long, painful, stressful period of life that will last many months through football season and Christmas and far into the next year and beyond. We will be challenged beyond anything we have ever encountered. The most unacceptable reality is that I will have to live as long as eight or nine months without any breasts. What will I look like? What will Robert think? What will happen to our sex life? How will we get through all this? I haven't been biopsied yet, but I already assume that both breasts will be removed. What if there is no cancer in the left breast? With my history, should I have it removed anyway? Isn't it almost a certainty that I will develop cancer in the left breast eventually? Will I be right back here in a year or two? I absolutely cannot go through this again.

I decide that no matter what the results of the biopsy are, I will have a double mastectomy. I hate the thought of having no breasts, but I can't cope with the possibility of having a single reconstructed breast that doesn't match the other. I want to rid myself of both troublesome breasts that I have begun to detest as a threat to my life and my happiness. I want them replaced with breasts that are symmetrical and as natural looking and feeling as surgical techniques will allow.

Robert and I arrive home weary and disillusioned. There is nothing to do except try to absorb what is happening to our lives while we go about our normal routine. We decide to sit outside on the driveway like we so often do in the afternoon and talk. Robert waters the grass and feeds the birds in the backyard. We try to envision what will happen to us. We go to bed shortly after sunset. Some of my initial discouragement is beginning to wear off.

I go back to work on Thursday and Friday and am thankful for the wonderful distraction my work provides me. I see so many people during the day who have such greater concerns and problems that, in comparison, I feel blessed. On Saturday, I am apprehensive waiting for Jessica to return from her church trip. She arrives home at 12:30 A.M. I let her fix a snack, as teenagers must, then I tell her about all that has occurred while she was away. She is worried and has questions, but she is strong and accepting. Jessica has an extraordinary faith she lives every day. With her family history, she will have to be vigilant about breast self-examination and regular checkups. Maybe Jessica will one

21

day be able to live in a world free of this awful disease. Brooke and Jessica react in a supportive way, but I think they both are hiding their feelings from me. I am so sorry to bring this trauma into our home.

Sunday is Father's Day. Robert has called our pastor, Dr. Hugh Davis, and told him about me. Coincidentally, Hugh has arranged to hold a healing service after church for Jill Moneyhun, a good friend who has been diagnosed with lung cancer. Hugh asked Robert if we would like to be included, and Robert said yes without asking me. As a Methodist, I have never been to a healing service and don't know what to expect. I am very nervous about going to church this Sunday because I know the news is getting out. I am also a bit anxious about the idea of a healing service. I hope there will be a few prayers in typical Methodist fashion, and we will be on our way. I am wrong.

Robert and I walk nervously into the education building at Martha Bowman Memorial United Methodist Church and encounter the bulletin board listing the Circle of Concern. There in bright red letters is my name. Oh no, I think. I don't want my name on that list, even though I so appreciate the love in my church. In a moment or two we run into friends coming out of Sunday School and learn that I am half dead and it is only a matter of time. I see my dear friend, Sandra Crisp, and the tears flow. I decide to turn around and go home. This is not what I want, and it is not what I need. But Sandra, bless her, hugs me, and we are able to stop crying and even laugh a little. I manage to build up the courage to go into the sanctuary.

Robert and I sit in our usual pew to the left of the pulpit and are joined by Brooke, Leah, and Jessica. I feel terribly self-conscious as if everyone is whispering about me. I want to stand up and shout, "Yes, I have breast cancer, but I have no intention whatsoever of dying— certainly not before the Georgia Bulldawgs once again whip Florida."

Several friends come over and speak to me and offer their prayers. The service is spirit-filled. When Hugh comes to the part where he reads off the names of those in the Circle of Concern, for some reason, he calls me "Robbie" instead of Rorie. Maybe nobody knows who that is, I hope. I feel a welcome sigh of relief.

After the service, we all stay with Jill and her husband, Wally, and their family. About a dozen members of the church remain with us in front of the altar. The healing service is begun by our associate pastor,

John Mitchell, who is very serious and removes his shoes as a symbol of reverence for where we are and what we are about to do. John has a big hole in his sock, which strikes me as being funny under the circumstances. Hugh follows John's example and takes off his shoes; he has a hole in his sock, too. They both pray and anoint Jill's head with oil and then mine as we kneel holding on to each other. Then our families and friends lay their hands on us. Hugh almost shakes because he is so moved by the Holy Spirit. I know Jesus is standing right there behind Hugh and John as I am overcome by the most loving and warm sense of peace. Robert's eyes fill with tears, and my family hugs me and each other. Everyone hugs me and Jill and Wally. We all know that healing has truly taken place.

Are our cancers gone? No, I still have breast cancer, and Jill still has lung cancer. But we have a deep conviction about God's greater version of healing that embraces the spirit and assures us of everlasting life. While our bodies still have this fearful disease, our souls are healed, and Jill and I gain what I now understand as blessed assurance.

Reflecting on that service, I realize that we all have holes in our socks. I would have never known that John and Hugh had holes in their socks unless they were willing to come before God and ask that He accept us as we really are. Some of us may have cancer; some of us may have lost our will to live; some of us may feel the pain of failure, loneliness, or sin. No matter how successful or prosperous or in control of life we may appear, no matter how much we have been possessed by our troubles, all of us have holes in our socks. And all of us need Jesus.

My family is able to release a great deal of emotion that has been building up for several days. We leave the church on a spiritual high. I don't want to go home, so Robert takes all of us to Applebee's for lunch. While we are sitting there engaged in light conversation, I have the strangest feeling that none of this is real. I am caught up in a dream, and soon I will wake up. Someone else is having a biopsy tomorrow. Not me. This doesn't happen to me.

I go to bed early and wake up at 2:00 A.M., my mind churning. Panic always waits in the dead of night and lunges at me during the most quiet and still moments. I pray for the feeling of peace I had earlier in the day, but it is slow in coming. I drift back to sleep around

6:00 A.M. and get up an hour later. I am not as nervous as perhaps I should be. Everyone who will take care of me today is a friend. I'll be in Outpatient Holding where I work, and I will get special care from my friends. I'll wear a sassy turquoise shorts outfit that will help me feel good. My sweet Greek friend, Aleca, our medical receptionist, greets me and hugs me and Robert. My nurse friends Deborah, Cheryl, Angela, and Kim surround me with hugs. I'm assigned to Room 8. I change into my hospital gown and am given a little Valium, which is very relaxing. Robert and Jessica are hovering around me. Brooke and Leah will arrive later.

The procedure is called a marking mammogram. Dr. Dale needs to be as precise as possible. The radiologist actually creates a roadmap of sorts for the surgery. I am wheelchaired over to Radiology and keep passing by friends and co-workers. Many haven't heard about me yet. They ask what's going on, and I joke that I'm a Mystery Shopper and they better treat me well. Everyone laughs, but I see concern in their eyes. Dear Lord, keep me smiling, I pray silently as I'm pushed through the hallways.

A marking mammogram is not a pleasant experience. The breast is squeezed between two metal plates, and the radiologist inserts a small needle into the suspicious area. It's uncomfortable but not unbearable. The procedure lasts about forty-five minutes. I see more co-workers in Radiology who have seen my films and know what's going on. They also look at me with concern.

I am wheeled back to Room 8, and my handsome Jamaican anesthesiologist, Dr. Alrick Brooks, comes in to start my IV. He is startled that his patient this morning is me. He gives me a hug and tries to reassure me. Brooke and Leah come in, and in a moment Dr. Dale comes by to explain what will happen and how long it will take. I'm wheeled down the hall on a stretcher to the OR. I'm surprisingly calm and relaxed. Patients pass by me all day long on this short journey, but today is my first experience looking up at faces staring down at me as the ceiling lights pass by in an eerie procession. I think to myself that every doctor and nurse should be a patient in the area they work in order to better understand how their patients feel.

With one quick shift, I'm moved from the stretcher onto the small OR bed. Immediately, the staff starts hooking me up to all the impressive monitoring equipment. This has to be terribly frightening to someone who doesn't understand what's going on. I asked for David Littleton to be my nurse anesthetist, and he is waiting on me with some terrific medicine, which enables me to go in and out of light sleep and talk throughout the biopsy. I have no sensation of pain, but I am aware of movement around me. Then I'm in the Recovery Room, and I hear the constant beeps from monitoring equipment and conversations going on around the other beds. My nurse and attendant buddies cater to me, giving me a heating tube under my blanket and a welcome cold drink. Robert comes in and looks relieved to see me propped up and talking to everyone. Jessica, Brooke, and Leah come in for a short visit, and then I'm back in Room 8.

Dr. Dale comes into the room and has changed his mind from the initial plan to proceed with mastectomies. He has found a large tumor and believes that some chemotherapy will be necessary to shrink the mass before surgery. He says he will be able to get a much better result if the tumor is smaller. I have an appointment with Dr. Fred Schnell, an oncologist, for the next afternoon. Robert has known Dr. Schnell for years, and there is no question which oncologist we want to see. I love putting my turquoise outfit back on and heading home.

The next day Jessica comes to the Medical Center to accompany me to the doctor's office. When it is time to go, my friend Angela hugs me, and I start crying. She assures me I'll be okay. Jessica and I go by Robert's office, and we all walk to the oncologist's office together, arriving at 2:30 P.M. It is a stifling hot June day. We enter the large suite of offices for four oncologists just a block down the street from the Medical Center. After a few minutes in a packed waiting room, we are escorted into the patient care area where we see big comfortable reclining chairs in every corner. I detect a peculiar smell and quickly decide this is not a place I want to be. In one chair sits an older man with a tube going into a vein in his left hand. His eyes are half closed, he has no hair, and his skin is ashen gray. He looks very ill and alone. I don't want to be alone during chemotherapy, and I know I won't be. I'm surprised that patients all sit around in a big room together for chemotherapy. Frankly, I envisioned being in a private room and maybe even on a bed. As a nurse, I probably should know more about all this, but I don't deal with chemotherapy, so I am as naive as anyone.

Robert, Jessica, and I sit in a nicely decorated examining room. A nurse asks me lots of questions while filling out another one of those endless forms. She is friendly and has a warm sense of humor. I don't know Dr. Schnell as well as Robert does, and I don't know what to expect. In a few minutes he comes in. I immediately think he looks like Harrison Ford. He has beautiful deep eyes that look straight through me. I have this picture flash across my mind that I'm talking to Indiana Jones. Maybe I'm trying to find something to take my mind off the reason I'm here.

Dr. Schnell says hello to Jessica and tells us it is difficult when a patient is someone he knows personally, but he needs to go down the list of things to cover so nothing is overlooked. He knows he has to manage his feelings and be sure we are treated the way he treats all his patients. We give him our absolute approval. He stops talking as he looks intently at my records, then Robert and Jessica leave the room for a few minutes while he examines me. I have stitches and some minor swelling from the biopsy on the side of my left breast. There is the beginning of some bruising on both breasts from the biopsy and marking mammogram.

Robert and Jessica return. I assure Dr. Schnell that he can talk freely in front of Jessica. This bright sixteen-year-old is getting an education in reality that may save her life one day. This is a large tumor, and I have a swollen lymph node in my axillary region with a significant ulcer on the right breast. Dr. Schnell carefully explains the four stages of breast cancer in very understandable language. A Stage I cancer means the cancer cells have not spread beyond the breast, and the tumor is less than 2 centimeters across. Stage II means the cancer has invaded the underarm lymph nodes, or the tumor is between 2 and 5 centimeters across or both. Stage III means the tumor is more than 5 centimeters, and there is direct skin involvement, ulceration, and lymph node invasion. It is referred to as locally advanced cancer. Stage IV is metastatic cancer, meaning the cancer has gone from the breast through the lymph nodes and is invading other parts of the body. I'm convinced Dr. Schnell is leading up to telling me I have Stage IV. I'm relieved to hear him say I have a locally advanced carcinoma. Imagine being thankful about having a Stage III cancer. I have to place everything into perspective. I know that as bad as this diagnosis is, it could be worse. . . . Today is the 18th day of June, 1996. Robert and I were sitting on the beach watching that beautiful sunset just nine days ago.

What are my options? I can participate in a study on the efficacy of bone marrow stem cell replacement or else undergo a more conventional chemotherapy regimen. The stem cell study sounds more complicated and more expensive, although it is covered by insurance. I wonder how anyone ever goes through all this without adequate health insurance. How fortunate Robert and I are to have good insurance. Dr. Schnell puts no pressure on me to participate in the study and is straightforward about the fact that one approach has not proven any more effective than the other. I choose chemotherapy and will come to the office once every three weeks and have three drugs administered intravenously over a couple of hours. I am informed that one of the drugs can be a burden to the heart, and I must first have a heart scan. I have an appointment to return to the Regional Imaging Center on Friday afternoon. I've already encountered an obstetrician/gynecologist, radiologist, oncological surgeon, oncologist, pathologist, and anesthesiologist—and my treatment hasn't even begun.

My mind is filled with thousands of images racing by like a videotape on fast forward. How sick am I going to get? I've heard so many horror stories. And what about my hair? I cannot lose my hair. Maybe I'll be the exception. Not everyone loses their hair, I tell myself. I can accept a mastectomy, but not losing my hair. Robert will not only have a wife with no breasts but with no hair. Oh God, is this really happening to me?

I am so tired and need the rest of the week off. The heart scan on Friday proves that I can proceed with chemotherapy, so my first session is scheduled for the next Thursday. Robert and I desperately need a normal weekend where we sit outside and cook out and enjoy our family. Thank goodness there is good weather so Robert can do some yard work. He tells me he does his best thinking when he's mowing the grass and watering, and there will be plenty of opportunity for that the next few days. We go to church, where many people come up to me and tell me they are praying for and thinking about me. My name is now in the weekly bulletin and will probably be there for many, many months. The weekend provides some rest and the illusion of freedom from this disease that is imprisoning me. But I cannot escape from the concerns I have about my ability to tolerate chemotherapy and its side effects.

Back at work, I am thankful that I feel well and my hours are filled with the normal flow of patients and their families. My friends are acting peculiar and are ducking around corners and hiding behind doors and whispering. I know something is up, but don't know what to expect. I think I'm a good detective and decide that they're going to have a surprise lunch. Jessica comes by for lunch, and no one objects to our leaving for the cafeteria, so my theory proves wrong.

When we return, I'm ushered back into an empty patient room. Sitting on the stretcher is the most beautiful, huge basket of presents I have ever seen. There are bath oils, lotions, soaps, sexy nighties, inspirational books, candles, candy, perfume, wine, and stacks of other presents too large for the basket. Sitting in the middle of all these delightful gifts is a big red Elmo doll and a videotape on Big Red Fire Engines. The girls tease me about my attraction to firemen and fire engines. They call me 911 Rorie because I'm the first one to hear a siren and always want to rush down to the Emergency Center anytime a fire engine comes to the Medical Center. These wonderful friends have been working behind the scenes for days collecting gifts and cards for me. I am elated by the love they express. I know I have some difficulties facing me in chemotherapy, but I am strengthened by the powerful sense of caring I feel surrounding me. God is so evident through little miracles. I am confident that God and my family and friends will be the anchors I so need to get me through my treatment. I will be ready.

From Robert. . .

We are sitting at the kitchen table when Dr. Luhrs calls about Rorie's suspicious mammogram. Dr. Luhrs has already made an appointment with Dr. Paul Dale for Wednesday morning. I don't want to go to work on Tuesday, but I do and have very little memory of anything that occurs that day. I know I won't say anything to anybody about Rorie. There will be plenty of time for that later.

When I wake up on Wednesday, Rorie is already dressed and downstairs. I have been extremely upset for days, but I am outwardly calm and confident. When I get into the shower I feel strange and gag over and over, even though I have an empty stomach. I can't stand the thought that Rorie is probably going to have at least one breast removed. The idea is so foreign to anything in our lives up to this point that my emotions are making me physically sick.

I'm glad that Rorie's appointment is with Paul Dale. He is a graduate of our surgery residency program and went to Los Angeles for additional specialized training in surgical oncology at the John Wayne Cancer Institute. He is involved in research and continues to publish his findings. I have great appreciation for a physician who is both a clinician and a researcher. Soon Rorie and I find ourselves in the examining room. I stay during her examination. Dr. Dale talks with us like a concerned friend. I am very pleased that a graduate of one of our residency programs learned that compassion is a vital part of competence.

I feel so sorry for Rorie as she can no longer hide the ulcer she has tried to cover up for months. There is no question about cancer in Rorie's right breast, but now the concern is about the left breast. I realize we are facing a double mastectomy. I cannot believe I'm sitting in a doctor's office listening to the probability of my wife losing both her breasts. And how serious, really, is the cancer in her right breast? Her right breast has to be removed, of course, but her left breast looks perfect. Can't it be saved? What about a lumpectomy? Is Rorie making the best decision about giving up what looks like a perfectly good breast? Is she going to be all right? What if the cancer has spread beyond her breast? How can doctors be sure that a Stage III cancer hasn't progressed to a Stage IV? Women die of breast cancer every day—lots of them. What is happening to us?

A million questions are flying through my mind, but Rorie is calm. I'll never forget her expression as long as I live. When Dr. Dale says he is sure she has cancer, Rorie doesn't blink. She just looks at me as though to say she is going to be fine and she doesn't want me to worry. She doesn't say anything, but when people are married for as long as we are, just a look is often enough. Her expression reflects her incredible character in which she is always concerned first about her children and me. I'm almost ashamed of myself for being so upset. I wish I had Rorie's strength and faith.

When we leave the office, Rorie and I return to work. I am experiencing a rush of adrenaline and feel like I'm in a mild state of shock at the same time. I walk into the medical education area in the West Tower of the Medical Center and ask Faye Payne, my graduate medical education coordinator, to come into my office. I close my door, which is unusual, and find it difficult to talk. Faye knows me well, and she sees I am struggling to keep from crying. I tell her that Rorie has cancer, and we sit down for a few minutes and talk. I fill her in on all I know so far and ask her to tell Terri, Melinda, and Adrianne who work in medical student and continuing medical education. These are all my closest friends whom I work with every day, but I cannot tell them individually. I just cannot do it.

I start to think about whom I should tell. I know that Rorie and I have to see Dr. Roy Powell at 4:00 P.M. I have to get out of the office immediately, so I go for a short walk outside the West Tower down in front of the Medical Center to the corner and turn around and come in the door by the cafeteria. I pass by people I see every day. I try to smile and realize that none of them know what is happening to me and my family. I don't want to talk to anyone yet, but I know I have to tell my boss who has become a good friend.

Fortunately, Dr. Louis Goolsby, our Senior Vice President for Medical Affairs, is in his office. I tell him Rorie has breast cancer, and we sit and talk for a few minutes as he offers me encouragement. He is very familiar with breast cancer in his role as an obstetrician/gynecologist and gives me a wonderful book on breast cancer that has pictures of women who have undergone mastectomies followed by breast reconstruction. It is helpful talking with Louis. I can't remember what I say, but I want him to know that I'm not going to let this stress interfere with my work. I'm not sure how much I can cope with. I really just want to take some leave and use all my vacation time right away. But this is a critical time in my career with a recent promotion, and I can't afford to let anything affect my responsibilities.

Back in the office I'm sure Faye has told everyone, but they know it's not yet time to say anything. Maybe tomorrow I'll be able to handle it. After an incredibly long day, it's finally time to leave to see another surgeon. I'm so thankful that Rorie and I are part of a medical community where we know so many people. Dr. Powell examines Rorie and measures the tumor. I think that determining the size of a tumor must be quite complicated and am surprised when he takes out a small ruler and places it against the lumpy part of the breast. He tells us about three different approaches to breast reconstruction. Rorie likes the idea about a procedure that eliminates much of the fat in the stomach area with a reduction in the inches around the waist. Roy warns us that she won't be able to do any sit-ups ever again, and we chuckle a bit when Rorie confesses that she isn't familiar with the concept of sit-ups.

We both go to work the next day. I start thinking about people I should call and write to. I'm not ready to talk, so writing is the best option. I have a painful knot in my stomach. I realize that I haven't yet cried. I've had lots of tears, but nothing like a good cry. Much of what is going on still feels like a bad dream, and I don't cry in dreams.

I sit down at my computer and write kind of a short, matter-of-fact letter I'll send to most of our friends. Rorie still hasn't told her mother or her sister, Debby, and I haven't contacted my sister, Nancy, in Jacksonville. First things first, I think, and I want to get this letter in the mail now. It will take a different approach telling our relatives. In the letter I mention a mastectomy and make it sound imminent because that is what I believe. I fax a copy to my close friend Ed Hagan at the Florida Medical Association where I used to work and send a copy to Bob Seligson, another close friend at the North Carolina Medical Society. I send more copies to Bulldawg friends who tailgate with us, including Bob and Ginny Manley and Jack and Josey Reid in Atlanta. Writing the letter helps me feel better, so I start to make some calls to friends in Macon. I have felt so alone the past couple of weeks; now I need my friends to know that I need them. I hate this sickening feeling of being all alone.

I call the dean of the medical school, Dr. Doug Skelton, and he is quite concerned as he knows Rorie very well. I call Mildred Howard, another good friend, and ask her to tell her husband Bob, and then I call Jessica's godmother, Paula Wingers. I call Ray Davis, the president of Rorie's high school class and one of my college fraternity brothers who now lives in Atlanta. Ray isn't home, so I speak with his wife,

Darlene. I know Ray will call the instant he hears the news, and he does. I instinctively call several of my best friends, including Judge Bill Self, Jimmy Taylor, and Pat Meyer. In the next day or two I will get in touch with Joe Sandefur and Ronnie Rowe. I send letters to old friends in the Florida Medical Association, including Dr. Dan Nunn and Dr. Yank Coble and my best friend in high school, Don Davidson, who lives in Jacksonville. After addressing a stack of letters and making several telephone calls, I have had enough for today.

Rorie and I cook out tonight, and Paula Wingers comes over. The minute Rorie sees Paula, she begins to cry. They hug each other and talk about what will happen next. Paula will ask members of Forest Hills United Methodist Church to start praying for Rorie. It's important that Paula, of all people, comes by tonight. She was there when Jessica was born and has always remembered our daughter on her birthday and at Christmas. Today is the beginning of a series of telephone calls and cards that start pouring in for Rorie. I begin to sense God working in our lives as the love for Rorie becomes more and more evident.

On Friday I'm responsible for our annual retreat for new chief residents. This involves our residency program directors and those residents who will serve as chief residents in the new academic year. No one mentions Rorie, so I assume no one knows. My mind is preoccupied, but I'm told I did a good job and this is the best retreat we've had so far. I want the day to end. I want to go home. I am so tired.

It's Saturday. For some reason I don't understand, I find it very difficult to call Hugh Davis, our minister. I love Hugh and need him, but I'm afraid I may get too emotional as the events of the previous week are tearing away at my composure. I feel as if I'm about to explode. His wife Becky answers and has to call him in from cutting the grass. Hugh says all the comforting words I knew he would and invites Rorie and me to join a healing service the next day for Jill, a friend who has lung cancer. Without hesitating, I say yes, not knowing what it will involve nor how Rorie will react. Then I call my dear friend Joe Sandefur. He struggles for something to say. I feel terrible having to tell him, knowing that I will probably ruin his day.

Later this afternoon I exercise to try to rid myself of some tension, and then I take a shower. Finally, all alone, I break down and cry. It is the kind of weeping that rages through my whole body in an uncontrollable burst of emotion and anger. Why does this have to happen to Rorie? And why does this have to happen to me? I'm very frightened and very angry. I haven't cried like this since my mother died in 1974. The noise from the shower prevents anyone from hearing me, and no one knows. I get myself dressed and go downstairs acting as if I'm just fine. I am hugging and kissing Rorie more than usual and wonder if I'm overdoing my attention. I know she appreciates it, but it may send her a signal that I'm worried.

I urge Rorie to call her mother. It has to be done, even though it will be the most difficult call. Once it's over, she will feel much better, I promise her. After several false starts, Rorie pours herself a glass of white wine and picks up the receiver. One reason Rorie has waited is because Jessica's choir tour left Panama City and went to Jacksonville to sing at a homeless shelter and Jessica stayed with her grandmother. So Rorie wants to be absolutely sure Jessica has left for Macon before calling. I go outside to water the grass because I know Rorie wants to be alone when she talks to Mary. Mary is eighty-three and a veteran of World War II, an army nurse who served in Patton's 3rd Army. She is the only parent we have left since both my parents are gone as well as Rorie's father. Mary tells Rorie that it should be her with cancer, not her child. Grandma is extraordinarily strong and healthy, but this news has to be devastating.

Sunday is my day to usher at church. I have to almost drag Rorie into the sanctuary after she sees her name in the Circle of Concern. I know she hates this. After church we stay for the healing service. Now Rorie and I and Brooke and Jessica are able to start the healing process. I weep, and Brooke weeps, and we hug each other for the first time in years. God has so many messages for us this day, and I can see we will learn lessons from this painful experience. Already I feel God telling me to show more affection to my son and to be a better father and a better friend. I hear Hugh proclaim to Rorie that she is forgiven and healed, and I understand that healing has many dimensions. I realize that healing is always there for us if we are only willing to embrace its true meaning. I see Rorie beaming with faith. I see a glimpse of God in her face. She is His child, and He will not let her go through cancer alone. I see her laugh about John and Hugh both having holes in their socks. I slowly open up to God's message that I don't have to be perfect and it's all right to hurt and be afraid and angry. I don't have to be strong all the time, and I'm not letting Rorie down if I have some kinks in my armor and holes in my socks.

Monday morning brings the big day. Rorie is everyone's cheerleader. I find it ironic that Rorie is assigned to Room 8 in Outpatient Holding because I was in the same room about a year earlier when I had a procedure to stretch my esophagus. I was having trouble swallowing and had a common procedure called an esophageal dilatation. Rorie was my nurse that day. She started my IV and was there with me in Recovery when the Versed wore off. Now the nurse is the patient.

Everyone around here seems to love Rorie. As she's wheeled down the hallway, many of her co-workers are startled at seeing her and don't know what's going on. I walk along following the stretcher for as far as I'm allowed, and then it's time to wait. Brooke and Leah have joined me and Jessica, and I take everyone downstairs to the cafeteria. It is too early for lunch and too late for breakfast, but there doesn't seem to be anything else to do. I have a couple of bites out of a salad and sit without much to say while the kids have something to eat. Then we walk up one flight of stairs and go to the Gift Garden and look around, and then it's back up to Room 8. Only an hour has gone by, but it feels like half a day. One of Rorie's nurse buddies comes in and says I can come down to Recovery. When I enter, Dr. Brooks, her anesthesiologist, greets me and reports that the patient is fine. She is wide awake and says she is in very little pain and the whole thing was a "piece of cake."

When Rorie is taken back to her room, Dr. Dale comes in and says the tumor is quite large and needs to be reduced by chemotherapy. The plan for an immediate mastectomy is changed because operating now would take so much tissue that a skin graft would be required. The idea of radiation is also brought up and sounds like a necessary follow-up to surgery. At this point there is still no definitive diagnosis of cancer in the left breast. We will have to wait for that report, and it might be several days.

When we arrive home, there are five cards in the mail. Cards are arriving every day, proving that most of our friends have heard the news. When we meet with Dr. Schnell, we learn that chemotherapy is an absolute must regardless of the result of the left breast biopsy. The left breast is the least of our worries. Fred proposes that Rorie participate in a clinical study where bone marrow cells are extracted and later transfused back into the body. Rorie wants the more traditional approach to chemotherapy that will involve a session every three weeks for 12 to 15 weeks. When the tumor appears to stop shrinking, the treatment will stop. Rorie decides to take the rest of the week off.

It's Thursday. I'm at work and feel like I'm walking around in a funk. I am getting calls each day, and friends at the Medical Center are asking me about Rorie. I'm so glad she stays home to get some rest today. She and Jessica decide to drive the twenty minutes up the road to Juliette, Georgia, for lunch at the Whistle Stop Cafe. This is the setting for the movie *Fried Green Tomatoes.* We love the story, and this haunting little town has taken on special meaning for us. Before they leave, Rorie discards the biopsy bra for one of her own. There may be less support, but it's more comfortable, she tells me.

I know everyone is concerned about Rorie and me, but it's getting tiring answering the same questions over and over. I find that people fall into two categories. They either want lots of details, or they say absolutely nothing. There are people who work very close with me who can't help but know about Rorie, yet they haven't said a word. I realize everyone has their own way to deal with a life-threatening illness. I never used the word "cancer" with Rorie, and I know that some of my friends have to cope with Rorie's diagnosis through silence. Our friends and relatives want to help, but it's Rorie and I who have to find a way to live with this problem. We feel the prayers all around us, which is what we need most.

On Friday, Rorie's number-one companion, Jessica, goes with her for the heart scan. I feel sorry for Jessica. She should be enjoying the summer before her senior year in high school, but she has the burden of her mother's cancer. She wants to know all the facts and to hear what each doctor has to say. God bless you, Jessica. You are a source of great strength for your mother.

After the heart scan, I take the whole family out to lunch at the Green Jacket. This is a welcome treat, and everyone is in high spirits. Something as simple as going out to lunch has taken on much more importance. I seem to notice little things more often these days. All of a sudden each morning I've started to feed the birds, squirrels, and a feisty chipmunk in my backyard. We've got two old tree stumps behind the kitchen window, and my critter friends wait for me to pour a pile of bird seed or peanuts. I've expanded the menu and learned that squirrels love strawberries and peaches but don't care much for bananas. I expect to discover a note one morning saying "Hold the Bananas." Anyway, this ritual has become very important to me as it reminds me of how precious life is and how there is so much around us we fail to see.

On Saturday, life appears to be quite normal. Rorie looks wonderful and is healthy except for the cancer in her breast—at least that's what I believe. We cook out as usual and have a giant stack of baby back ribs that have been soaking in root beer. We see the first lightning bug of the summer. I have trouble enjoying myself as much as I should, thinking that this pleasant evening is the calm before the storm of chemotherapy. Our Florida Gator friends, Mary Kay and Joey Samorisky, call from Jacksonville. They are very upset, but Rorie and I joke and laugh and act as if we're doing just great. I don't think our friends buy it.

It's awfully hot on Sunday morning, so I decide to forget the necktie and wear a golf shirt to church. Rorie's name is in the church bulletin for the first time; I fear it will be there for months. Church is good medicine. Hugh's sermon speaks directly to us. He talks about frogs and skunks and helps us chuckle about the need to ignore the skunks in our lives. You see, if you encounter a skunk and corner him, you know the result. But if you ignore him, he'll just go away. Boy, have we ever got a skunk in our lives!

This is a good day. Brooke and Leah come over, and we drive out to look over a new housing development called Westchester Hills. Rorie and I have dreamed about building a house ever since we got married. Like most couples, it just isn't possible while you have to buy school clothes and pay for braces. But we think we may be at a point in life where we can fulfill our twenty-five-year-old dream. We find the perfect lot on a cul-de-sac on Somersby Lane. We like the view and the name of the street. When we get home, we take out a pile of house plans we've collected from magazines. Brooke and Leah tell us their ideas about kitchens, closets, and garages. I am happy to see the look on Rorie's face as she talks about how she'd like her kitchen arranged. We're looking ahead, I think to myself. This is what Rorie needs. Is there a way we can do this? Will we ever end up on Somersby Lane?

The telephone rings. It's Dr. Bob Windom, former Assistant Secretary of Health under President Ronald Reagan. Bob is at an American Medical Association meeting in Chicago and has just heard about Rorie. We usually attend AMA meetings. This is the first one we've missed in several years. As soon as we hang up, Dr. Henry Yonge in Pensacola calls. He has just heard the news. It feels good to hear from so many people I worked with in the Florida Medical Association. This is the best day Rorie and I have had since Rorie had her mammogram seventeen days ago.

Rorie wakes up at 4:00 A.M. as usual on Monday and leaves for work before I get out of bed. When I arrive at 8:00 A.M., Dr. Jerry Tift is waiting for me in my office. Jerry is a pathologist and the chairman of our continuing medical education committee. He is very sorry about Rorie and tells me the pathology report indicates a common ductal carcinoma in the right breast and a less common tubular carcinoma in the left. I thank Jerry and go up to Outpatient Holding to tell Rorie who is not at all surprised to have cancer confirmed in the left breast. As far as chemotherapy, the regimen will be the same whether or not there is any cancer in the left breast.

Chemotherapy is a scary word. I should know better. After all, an aspirin is chemotherapy if you think about it. It's just that with cancer, it means a group of highly potent chemicals designed to attack and kill the cancer, often with side effects such as nausea and loss of hair. Cancer is the enemy, and we want to destroy the enemy. If there are some casualties along the way, for example, Rorie's pretty hair, so be it. It is so easy for me to talk tough.

Today, thirty-five new residents arrive for orientation. At lunch I'm expected to give a short welcome and pep talk as director of medical education. I talk from the heart. My emotions get the best of me as I share with them my wife's recent diagnosis and the fact that most of her doctors are associated with our medical education program. I tell them that medical education isn't just a job for me anymore. I want them to learn that hope is part of medicine. I urge them to learn as much as they can about human beings while they're learning about human bodies. These young doctors listen to me, and several continue to check with me on Rorie's progress.

Rorie's old high school friend, Ray Davis, called last week from Atlanta and is coming down to see us. This will be an important visit for Rorie and me as Ray shares many experiences with each of us. I have developed an appreciation for friends who make time and distance irrelevant. If you only see a true friend once a year or once a decade, it doesn't matter. The friendship is still there.

A long letter from my sister Nancy is waiting for us on top of a huge mountain of cards. She is shaken by the news of Rorie's cancer and is searching for something, anything she can do. Rorie and I feel so bad to know that our families and friends are suffering along with us. They may find it impossible to think of the right words; so do we.

Ray is coming tomorrow night. The house is a wreck. Rorie straightens up around the house. I should help, but I don't. When it's time for bed, she puts on her nightgown and mumbles something about no one helping her and breaks down and cries. In all our years together, she has never cried like this. Her weeping comes from deep in her soul. I see that the time has finally come to let out the anger and fear. I hold her as close as I can as we lie in bed together, trying to assure her that she needs to have these feelings and it's okay. I am so sorry this has happened, I whisper. I'm mad and afraid, too. But it's going to be all right, it's going to be all right. I have never felt so close to Rorie as I do these few moments. Soon the tenseness in her body fades away, and she falls into a deep sleep. She is exhausted.

In a few minutes I turn off the light. Though I have prayed every day, this time I kneel beside the bed and lay my hands on Rorie asking God to please protect her, to give her courage, and to lift her spirit away from the cancer in her body. I thank God for the enormous blessings we've had in our life together. I am surrounded by such stillness and a feeling of peace that I am able to sleep better than I have in months.

When I wake up, Rorie is already at work as usual. Arriving at my office, my direct extension is ringing. It's Rorie calling with confidence in her voice. She tells me she feels much better and sounds almost embarrassed for crying the night before. Both of us feel better. Dr. Skelton calls while attending the AMA meeting in Chicago, expecting Rorie to be in surgery having a mastectomy. He has not been informed that the plans have changed and chemotherapy will start Thursday. At lunch Rorie tells me she has called Dr. Schnell's office and asked the nurse for some Zofran and Ativan to help avoid nausea and also for a prescription for a hair prosthesis because it is time to start planning to lose her hair. I am encouraged to see her take charge of her care and want to get started with treatment.

More cards come in the mail today. We get at least one card every day. I know this will stop soon. Rorie is keeping every one. Perhaps the most meaningful card yet comes from Susan Bagwell. She is married to Dr. Tim Bagwell, our former minister. Susan and Tim have been going through exactly the same experience with breast cancer. Susan had a mastectomy, and then doctors found cancer in the other breast, and she had a second mastectomy. I remember the Sunday when Tim stood in front of the church and announced that Susan had cancer. We were so upset about what they were facing and never dreamed we would be in the same circumstance two years later. Susan's message to Rorie was powerful. She included a copy of the following, which we read over and over:

> *Cancer is limited . . .*
> *It cannot cripple love*
> *It cannot corrode faith*
> *It cannot eat away peace*
> *It cannot destroy confidence*
> *It cannot kill friendship*
> *It cannot shut out memories*
> *It cannot silence courage*
> *It cannot invade the soul*
> *It cannot reduce eternal life*
> *It cannot quench the Spirit*
> *It cannot lessen the power of the Resurrection.*

Susan's card and letter are messages from God. God is using her to help us. I am sure of that. The doorbell rings. It's Brenda Scherer, a nurse buddy. She brings us lasagna and dessert as a surprise. She doesn't know Ray is coming over, and, presto, we have dinner. I can tell Brenda loves Rorie. Her concern and love radiate from her face. Ray arrives at 7:00 P.M. This guy never ages. He must be Dick Clark. He looks the same as he did in high school thirty years ago. And he even *weighs* the same. It's just not fair. Ray walks down memory lane with Rorie and me while Brooke, Leah, and Jessica devour every story as we sit around the kitchen table. Ray and I swap old fraternity stories and trade a few lies, and everyone laughs about events that can't possibly be true. Rorie and Ray have their thirtieth high school reunion next summer. It is vitally important to Rorie to be there. Thank you Susan and Brenda and Ray. God sent all of you today, and you are a part of His plan to answer our prayers.

God must be working overtime. Wednesday is a day Rorie will cherish forever. Her friends in the Surgery Center give her a truckload of presents, which is a complete surprise. The love I see surrounding Rorie is overwhelming. It is heartfelt and sincere. So many things are happening that cannot be coincidence. An old friend of Rorie's from nursing school, Maria Louise, calls tonight. She hasn't seen Rorie in four years and doesn't know about the cancer. But tonight she calls. And I am pleased that Rorie has been reading my father's Bible every day. It occurred to me that Daddy died exactly twenty years ago today, June 26, 1976. I believe with all my heart that he has a new life in heaven. And I pray that tomorrow is the beginning of a new life for Rorie. This is the eve of chemotherapy, and it is a day of little miracles.

CHEMOTHERAPY
Accepting the Challenge

"Those of us here in Bulldog Country want you to know that you are in our thoughts and prayers as you begin treatment and move toward a full recovery."

—Vince Dooley

From Rorie . . .

Chemotherapy. I go to work today to keep my mind occupied, and I also need to earn as many personal leave and sick days as I can. I may have to be out many times the next few months, so I can't afford to miss work unless I am very sick. Jessica takes me to work so I won't have to think about driving home. I watch the clock all day. It doesn't want to move. Robert and I eat lunch together, and he tries to encourage me. At 2:00 P.M., Jessica returns and has my Elmo doll for good luck. I shed a few tears and tell my friends goodbye, and then Jessica and I walk downstairs to get Robert. He has promised to go with me to every chemotherapy session unless he's gone out of town at a meeting.

I have some mints and lemon drops in my pocket because I've heard chemotherapy can produce an unpleasant taste in your mouth. I am so scared. It is a typical blistering hot summer day in Macon as we walk the short block to Dr. Schnell's office. This is one of the longest walks of my life. We arrive and go almost immediately into the treatment area. All the nurses are smiling. I smile, too, even though I am afraid. Regina Goforth, a friend from church, is there with one of her friends who is on chemotherapy. Regina hugs me. I am so glad to see her. She is one of those special people who has already begun the process of becoming one of God's angels.

My nurse, Lynn, sits me in a big easy chair and assembles her equipment. Robert pulls a small chair over and sits as close as he can while Jessica sits in another easy chair. My little Elmo is in my lap, and I hold on to him tightly. Lynn is a talker. I like her. She talks to me as she hooks up the IV and looks straight into my eyes as she explains the side effects of the drugs she is about to administer. She says, "You *will* lose your hair." I have been prepared for that, I guess, but Lynn's statement is so definite and without any doubt that I have to keep myself from starting to cry. I have a vision of myself totally bald, and I hate it.

Lynn places a small butterfly needle in my right hand. I don't feel anything. Blood is drawn, and an antiemetic is administered to prevent nausea. I am relieved to be given Zofran as requested. The first medicine I'm given is Adriamycin, which turns my urine red. Robert is holding my hand. I feel fine so far. I'm given Adriamycin through what looks like a giant hypodermic needle. Then I am given Cytoxan from a bag, followed by 5-Fluorouracil, or 5-FU for short. I feel nothing unusual. There is no bad taste in my mouth and no nausea. After about an hour and a half, the slow drips are over, and the bags are empty. Lynn removes the needle. We are ready to go home.

I am told that my white blood count will drop in seven to fourteen days, and I will have to watch carefully for infection when I am in such a vulnerable condition. We make another appointment for exactly three weeks later when my white blood count should be back up. This one treatment is about $1,500. I am amazed to think what the total cost of all my cancer treatments will be. I have read that when we add up chemotherapy, surgery, radiation, physician fees, and hospital bills, we can expect close to $100,000. How can people with no insurance survive?

The sunshine feels good on my face when we walk outside. Though I feel drained from the day's tension, I feel good. We stop by Revco on the way home and pick up some Compazine tablets and suppositories just in case I do have some nausea. I keep expecting to feel bad, but nothing happens. We order dinner from Steak Out. I inhale my steak, baked potato, and salad. I take a long luxurious bubble bath using some of my new gifts, put on a new nightie, and climb into bed. I have been granted custody of the remote control tonight and have my trusty barf bucket by the side of the bed. I am prepared for any eventuality. Robert and I are taking tomorrow off because I assume I will be sick, and I don't want to be alone.

I feel like a guinea pig with everyone observing me waiting to see what happens. All the family members, including out kitty cat, Puss, come in and join me on the bed. I feel like I'm disappointing my audience by not getting sick yet, but we have a good time. Finally, I take my prescription sleeping pill and close my eyes. Sleep comes quickly, and I sleep very deeply.

Chemotherapy

On Friday, I wake up listening to the birds chirping near the bedroom window. I open the blinds to see a beautiful day. I feel fine and wonder when I am going to get sick. While I wait, I decide to have some coffee and a bagel. Robert joins me on the deck while we watch his critters munch on some peanuts and strawberries. "Let's go to the Whistle Stop Cafe" is Robert's invitation. I say, "Why not?"

There is not much of a crowd in Juliette today, so we have most of the shops to ourselves. We find some fabulous Georgia Bulldawg shirts with the face of the bulldawg on the front and his southern end on the back. We decide we will wear these to Athens for the Tennessee game. It will be cool weather, and these black shirts will feel good. Lunch is terrific, and I eat more than usual. Poor Robert forgets that the restaurant doesn't take credit cards, and he doesn't have enough cash to pay the bill. The nice lady at the cash register asks, "Where are you from, honey?" When he says Macon, she tells him to just mail a check. We appreciate the kindness and head for home thinking about the dinner that Brooke and Leah are going to prepare for us. Rather than get sick, I am thinking alot about food. Dinner includes squash casserole, macaroni and cheese, grilled chicken, and dressing. Food is still my friend, and I feel perfectly normal.

On Saturday, I start to feel unusually tired. I am drinking lots of water as I was instructed to do to prevent cystitis. I am constantly visiting the bathroom, but I seem to have avoided the nausea I was expecting. On Sunday night, I feel like cooking and prepare a fancy chicken dinner but am disappointed that I can only eat a few bites. I am not nauseated, but I have lost the appetite that was so strong on Friday. This is the worst day after my initial chemotherapy treatment, but I am thankful it is not as bad as it could be. I feel blessed and welcome bedtime.

Back at work on Monday I'm greeted as though I'm a long-lost friend. Everyone is surprised and thankful that I didn't have an awful weekend. I feel quite normal and relish my work. I love my patients who don't have any idea that I'm a cancer patient. It's refreshing because I don't have to answer their questions. I so appreciate everyone's prayers and sincere concern, but being the center of attention for this reason is a drain on my energy and a strain on my nerves.

The next few days are filled with routine events such as going to work and shopping. I continue to receive cards in the mail. We have an enjoyable 4th of July and go see the movie *Independence Day*. This is the first 4th of July in years that we're not at the beach. I miss the fireworks over the water. The holiday is on Thursday, and we get Friday off automatically. Robert and I take Monday off because I want to go to the mall and look for hats. I am worried that my hair will start falling out any day. In fact, I believe it is getting thinner already. I order an expensive wig from a hair salon that looks great in the catalog. When it arrives, it looks like a bird's nest and makes me look like an old-time country and western singer on a bad hair day. I also order two more wigs on my own. I am so vain. I do not want to be bald, and I don't want Robert to have a bald wife.

Tuesday is a very good day at work and extremely busy. The shock of my diagnosis is starting to wear off, and people around me are paying less attention as things start getting back to normal. Jessica has her senior pictures made today. I'm reminded of the day when I had mine made. Those thirty years since the summer of 1966 have gone by too fast. God has been so good to me, and the Holy Spirit has filled my heart and is the most powerful medicine I've had. I don't know why I've avoided nausea and feel so good, but I'm happy just to say, "Thank you God," and accept it.

Tonight as I take my hair down and get ready for bed, I notice an unusual amount of hair in my fingers and in the sink. I brush my fingers through my hair, daring it to come out, and I produce a handful. It's not coming out in clumps yet, but my worst dream is becoming a reality. I've been expecting this, but I'm not able to accept it. I sit on the bed and look at the strings of hair in my hand and cry. Robert holds on to me, and he cries some, too. This is such an awful reminder that, yes, I do have cancer and no matter how optimistic we try to be, there will be many horrible things happening to me from now until the day all this is over. My sweet Brooke comes in the room and tells me he loves me and holds on to me, too. I am so blessed to have these two strong men with me. I take a melatonin to sleep better. It usually helps, but tonight I cannot sleep.

Robert and I lie in bed fully awake. He tells me to do what I have to do. He means I should stay home if I want to, that I don't have to keep working. My hair is tied back because I think it might start coming out in clumps. I get out of bed at 4:30 A.M. and call in to tell them I will be coming in late. I have decided to get my hair cut very short this morning and want to find a wig I will feel comfortable wearing. I call my favorite hairdresser, Hamilton, who insists that his customers schedule appointments weeks and sometimes months ahead. But he tells me to come in at 11:00 A.M. Jessica goes with me. Hamilton has been trying to get me to try a really short hairdo for a couple of years. Today he gets his wish. He whispers questions to me about my condition, and we laugh and have a great visit. He is a friend and promises to do a great job when I finally get my hair back and want to do something different.

My hair looks great, but I know this look will last only a few days. Jessica and I find a wig store, and I try on several wigs. I end up buying a brown one and a blonde one. Now I have five wigs and am ready for life as a bald lady. The next day everyone likes my hair and wants to touch it, but I'm afraid someone will accidentally pull out a big clump. When I get home, Robert and I decide to go to Carraba's for dinner. I take the T-tops off my Camaro because this may be the last time I can feel wind blowing through my hair for a long time.

Saturday is the historic day when we get to see the Olympic torch pass through Macon. Robert, Jessica, Brooke, Leah, and I stand on the corner of 2nd Street and Mulberry downtown. It is so exciting. I get goosebumps. Jessica and I were in Greece when the flame was lit, and now we see it pass by in Macon. So much has happened to me since we were in Greece.

I dread going to work on Monday. My hair keeps coming out. I must finally wear a wig. I dread the looks and the questions, but think I might as well shock everyone. So I put on my blonde wig and reach for as much courage as I can muster. My friends understand and know the reason why I look so different from when they last saw me, but others look at me as if to say, "Who does she think she is?" My buddies, Bill and Carlos, come by and check on me throughout the day and give me encouragement.

My right breast is burning today. I assume the chemotherapy is busy at work attacking my tumor. I have so many questions about what is happening to my body. I start my period today right on time, but don't know how long my cycle will continue. I'm told it will probably stop and may never return.

I am wearing different wigs just about every day. I know it keeps people off balance. One day I have short frosted hair; the next day I have shoulder-length brown hair. I find that blondes do have more fun. I try not to let my feelings get hurt by the way a few people are insensitive and ask, "What have you gone and done to your hair?" It's as if I've done something wrong. Sometimes, depending on who it is and the situation, I lean over and tell them that I have on a wig and why. Their expressions are priceless.

I cannot wait to get home in the afternoon and take off my wig, which is hot and itchy. It has been exactly twenty days since I began chemotherapy. This is the end of my hair. I pull it out in clumps and decide I want no trace of it. Brooke finds Robert's Norelco and shaves me bald. I try still another wig that arrived in the mail. This will be my favorite, and Robert loves it. It is another blonde one and makes me look like Ann Jillian, an actress and famous breast cancer survivor. Robert wants me to put on my new black Bulldawg shirt and blonde wig for a photo opportunity. I feel kind of sexy and agree to put on my red high heels and pose for some pictures we can send to friends. I want them to know that I'm doing well. The pictures turn out great. It's fun. I feel lucky that I still feel attractive but wonder what I'm going to do when I no longer have any breasts.

It is a new sensation having no hair. When I sleep, it's as though I have Velcro on my head and I kind of peel off the pillow. I discover that Robert rubbing his fingers over my head is very sensual. Funny, I never thought of the top of my head as an erogenous zone, but I like it. My second chemotherapy session comes and goes with Robert and little Elmo with me. There is a room full of people with me receiving chemotherapy. We talk and have such deep understanding for each other. I still have no nausea. Dr. Schnell reports that the tumor has shrunk. I am elated. Something good is happening. The cancer that was advancing so aggressively has either been stopped in its tracks or, even better, forced into retreat.

July is relatively mild. Attention is on the Olympics. I can't stand to hear about the TWA Flight 800 crash or the bombing at the Olympics in Atlanta. The opening ceremonies are unforgettable, although I cannot keep myself awake to see the lighting of the torch. I still feel well, but I tire easily and fall asleep quickly if I lie down on the couch.

I have many things on my mind that keep me from dwelling on my cancer. Jessica is representing Macon in the Georgia Junior Miss Contest in August. Robert and I are determined to find a way we can buy our building lot. The new housing development is progressing, and we have our hearts set on one of the most ideal lots. The developer isn't accepting deposits yet, and we are concerned that someone else might beat us to the punch. We were the first to move into our present neighborhood, and we want to buy the first lot in this new area. Robert has a conference coming up in St. Simons, Georgia, and I will go with him. I look forward to sitting around the pool wearing my blonde wig and sunglasses. Time is starting to drag. I want to speed up my treatment. But everything must come in a certain order. First chemotherapy, then the mastectomies, then possibly radiation, and then finally I will be able to have reconstruction and move on with life.

When I got the results of my mammogram, Robert and I decided to start separate diaries. We will not share these with each other, at least for awhile, but we will chronicle what is happening from our different perspectives. The idea of a book emerges, and after several weeks we decide to read each other's thoughts. This is wonderfully therapeutic and helps us communicate. It is often easier to write down feelings than to verbalize them. Robert writes a draft of a first chapter and allows the family to read it. He is a talented writer and has always wanted to publish a book, although not under these circumstances.

Church is my salvation. On July 28, we have communion. Our new associate pastor, Kelly Crissman, makes communion a very personal and full-of-life experience for the congregation. I have no way of knowing, but I bet Kelly also has holes in his socks. He would appreciate what that means. Robert and I kneel and pray at the altar. I pray that he can have the same inner peace I have discovered. I see him full of turmoil and worry. I know my cancer is constantly on his mind. He seems to be under enormous pressure to keep his work going well while he has this added burden and strain at home. This is exactly what I did not want to happen. I don't want him to hurt because of me, but it is inevitable.

The St. Simons trip arrives. I reluctantly leave Jessica at home as she gets ready for her contest. On the other hand, I want to be alone with Robert. When we arrive, our room isn't ready, so he goes on to his workshop as I wait to check in. The King & Prince is one of our favorite places, and I find it restful and cozy. When I check in, I look at the ocean from our balcony and am consumed with sadness. I look down at the pool and see all the women with their skimpy swimsuits on and feel sorry for myself for not being able to go down there and jump in. I can't get my wig wet, and I sure can't go down there without it. I hate these feelings of self-pity that are prompted by little events I can never anticipate. I am glad Robert is tied up in meetings and isn't here to see me cry. Later we go to Mullet Bay for a romantic dinner and then return and make love as though it is our honeymoon. I cherish these moments but can't help feeling anxious about what our sexual relationship will be like the days following my mastectomies.

In the morning, Robert rolls over and announces he will play hooky from his morning meeting. We have breakfast in bed and later have lunch by the pool. The workshop is disappointing to Robert, who says he should be teaching it. That afternoon, the skies turn black. A wonderful thundering summer storm rolls in with high winds and sheets of rain. We watch this drama unfold from our third floor balcony. I am sure my father is helping to orchestrate this event from heaven. He loved storms, as Robert does. I know this is a special message and gift to us from my father, Smitty. When the weather subsides, we see a huge sandbar about 200 yards offshore where two teenage boys have gotten stranded in a kayak. They're not the least concerned and sit down by their cooler and enjoy the uniqueness of their predicament. Their problems will be solved when the tide comes in, so they relax knowing all will be well. That's what I have to do. I have to convince Robert that we will get off this sandbar we find ourselves on because God promises that the tide will soon return and rescue us. We have to relax and believe that all will be well.

Back at work on Monday, my friend Tony, who used to work in the Surgery Center, comes by for a visit and asks if he can cook something for me. The next day he brings the most mouthwatering ribs I have ever eaten. This week I return for my third chemotherapy session, which falls on our twenty-sixth wedding anniversary. Robert sends a dozen beautiful red roses to me in Outpatient Holding. The card tells me he loves me, and I know that is so very true. Dr. Schnell is out of town, so I am examined by one of his partners, Dr. Deaton, who is optimistic and tells me he thinks this might be my last session. The tumor is smaller and appears to have reached a point where it is no longer shrinking. More chemotherapy doesn't seem to be indicated. I have a reaction to the medicine. My vein turns red up my arm but subsides in about thirty minutes. There is no champagne and romantic dinner this anniversary, as Robert and I spend it holding hands in an oncologist's office.

Mom and my sister Debby and her daughter Alex come up for the Junior Miss Contest. Robert has Merry Maids clean the house before our guests arrive. We order Jessica's flowers and get ready to attend the first performance. We are so proud of Jessica. Everyone is relieved that she is fortunate enough to participate, but she does not win. In the morning I wear my blonde wig to breakfast. Debby cries because I look so strange to her, and it reminds her of the seriousness of my illness. She is worried about me, but I am sometimes short with her when she asks questions. She is only trying to find out what's happening to me. I should be more patient.

When our company leaves, I go see Dr. Dale, who tells me I will have recovered from chemotherapy enough to have double mastectomies on Wednesday, September 4. I will definitely have to have radiation on the right side after surgery because of the lymph node infiltration and the likelihood the cancer could have spread beyond the breast into the chest wall. Also, because of the radiation and the amount of skin I will lose on the right side, Dr. Dale thinks I will be quite a challenge for Dr. Powell and his reconstructive skills. I am very disappointed and discouraged to hear that I may have still more chemotherapy after radiation. It occurs to me that my hair will soon start to grow back, but more chemotherapy will mean I will lose it for a second time. I cannot even think about that now. Maybe Dr. Schnell will decide that I've had enough. That is my prayer.

My perfect plan for reconstruction keeps changing. Now I know for sure that I cannot possibly have reconstruction until well into the next year. After the second and third chemotherapy treatments, I have been having a metallic taste in my mouth. Often food has a peculiar flavor. The third session has left me feeling more tired and drained than usual. Apparently, all this medicine has a cumulative effect. My period starts and is extremely heavy as if my reproductive system is making one last heroic effort before shutting itself down forever.

My depression ebbs and flows, but I always have this sense that God is with me. I know that when I feel sorry for myself, God waits patiently for me and never allows me to drift too far from His limitless love. I can remember allowing my children to cry because, as a parent, I knew that they would survive and recover from their pain. Now my Heavenly Father knows I will survive and recover. He is preparing me for surgery where I will lose part of my femaleness, but I will have the courage to be confident that my identity is what God has created in my soul and not in the mirror. There continues to be a dramatic change in me physically, but my spirit is connected to God and those I love, and it gains strength every day.

From Robert . . .

It is the beginning of chemotherapy. Everyone in my office understands how important it is for me to leave work early and go with Rorie. As we walk down Hemlock Street, we wave to friends passing by and are convinced that none of them know where we are going. When we arrive at Dr. Schnell's office, we walk back into the patient care area, which is very busy. I see several people hooked up to IVs. I'm glad I'm able to stay with Rorie and sit next to her. Rorie's nurse is kind and very thorough in telling her about side effects and the need to be careful about infections when her white blood count hits bottom. I hold Rorie's hand. When the nurse tells her she will definitely lose her hair, I have to keep myself from reacting. Rorie's eyes tear up for a moment, and then she seems to accept the certainty of it all. I learn a new word, *alopecia,* which means hair loss.

The powerful medicine starts to fill Rorie's veins. I wonder where it all will go in her body. There seems to be so much. I don't know how she can tolerate it. Our friend Regina comes by and gives Rorie a little hug. Later we're glad to see Jill, the girl who received the healing service with us. Jill looks tired, but she smiles and encourages us. Her hair has come back nicely. I say a quiet prayer that she is on the way to recovery.

I look around the room at the patients and feel Rorie's hand in mine and find it hard to believe that I'm sitting here with my beautiful bride as she undergoes chemotherapy for breast cancer. Rorie gets tearful as she squeezes my hand and tells Jessica and me how much she loves us. I want Rorie to know how much I love her, but I guess just being with her at this place and time may be enough. I can't help but start going through a mental list of all the terrible things that can happen to a couple in their marriage. I can remember as a young man of twenty-one or twenty-two, I couldn't imagine being married and then having to face breast cancer and my wife losing her breasts. It was incomprehensible. Now that event has arrived. In many ways, if this had to happen, I'm glad I'm older and more mature with a broader perspective. I don't know if I could have handled this situation as a very young man.

My thoughts take me back years as I relive the milestones in our life together. I recall our wedding day and our fifth anniversary when we renewed our vows in the same church with our parents standing with us. I recall the torturously long Sunday when Brooke was born in St. Vincent's hospital, the same place where I was born and both my parents died. I remember our trip to Athens when I was interviewed for my doctoral program and what a rainy night in Georgia that was. I remember being in the delivery room watching Jessica enter the world and be placed on Rorie's stomach as we both cried in joy. Most of my life's memories include Rorie.

One of my favorite songs is "How Do You Keep The Music Playing?" sung by James Ingram and Patti Austin. The lyrics, which I have grown to love, ask:

How do you keep the music playing?
How do you make it last?
How do you keep the song from fading too fast?
How do you lose yourself to someone, and never lose your way?
How do you not run out of new things to say?

Then it goes on to promise:

> *If we can be the best of lovers, yet be the best of friends,*
> *If we can try with everyday to make it better as it grows,*
> *With any luck, then I suppose, the music never ends.*

I have listened to that song hundreds of times driving home from work in recent weeks.

I'm so afraid. I don't want the music to end. I hate being here in an oncologist's office, and I hate Rorie's cancer, and I wish I could wake up from this nightmare. As cancer has consumed more and more of our lives, I am becoming more sensitive to what people have to say. I know I shouldn't do this, but I run kind of a tab on what people say, and I make what is probably an unfair judgment. But it's amazing the difference in people's reactions. Some offer great encouragement, while others want to tell me how tough it's all going to be. I think I'm starting to get the message about how tough it's going to be. What I want to hear is that my wife isn't going to die and she's going to get well and return to the life we built together.

After the first treatment is over, we go home expecting the worst. Rorie takes a bath with peach bubble bath, then puts on a pink nightie to match our new pink sheets and pink comforter. Jessica gives her a foot massage with peach lotion. Tonight, Rorie is truly a Georgia peach. She feels fine and looks forward to watching "ER" on television and viewing her Big Red Fire Engines tape. Another dear friend, Joe Orr, calls from Atlanta. His wife, Nancy, is hesitant to talk because she thinks she might get too emotional, but Rorie insists on talking to her and puts her fears at ease. Rorie doesn't get sick. She falls into a deep sleep. Good night, my love. God bless you and protect you. And may God give me strength.

The church bulletin arrives. Rorie's name has moved to the top of the list. This is the big day we hear so much about. It's the day after chemotherapy. But Rorie wakes up feeling energetic. We go to the Whistle Stop Cafe where the post-chemo patient eats barbecue ribs, cornbread, peach cobbler, and a fried green tomato. I send my sister a postcard photo of the cafe. Jessica hasn't seen the building lot we want to buy, so we drive by on the way home. Rorie pulls a leaf off an oak tree on the property and, with a little prayer, places it in her Bible. We will need divine intervention if we end up building a house on Somersby Lane.

That night the family sits outside. The moon is bright and full. Rorie tells me how she looked at that moon a few months before while in Greece, and she would pray about me back in Macon. She was so worried about cancer on that trip, and I was home counting the days until she returned when there would have to be a mammogram. I thought this would be one of the worst days of our lives, but it is one of the best.

At church, Rorie tells me she feels self-conscious as if people are wondering if she's lost weight, or what stage her cancer is in, or if her hair is thinning. It continues to be interesting how people react. One friend comes up to me and tells me he just heard about Rorie's problem. He doesn't say cancer. If Rorie had suffered a heart attack, he would have referred to a heart attack, but we still fear cancer so much that we don't even want to say the word. After church, Jessica asks me to go with her to buy a CD. I welcome our time together. Just a few weeks earlier I would have said I was too busy. But now every minute has become much more valuable.

Rorie goes to work and completes her ten-hour shift with no problems. She tells me she sometimes feels toxic. I am unable to fully appreciate what that must be like. We have our first week with no doctors, no examinations, no chemotherapy. What a relief! We receive a note from Jack and Josey, our Bulldawg friends in Atlanta, and Dr. Yank Coble sends a warm letter. His wife, Ohlyne, has been struggling with cancer for a very long time. They have a special understanding about what is happening to us.

One day after work, I meet with Rob Ballard, a local builder, because I want him to give me an opinion on the lot. Rob tells me it's a 10 on a 10-point scale. Rorie and I become more determined than ever. Rob and his wife, Penny, have a daughter fighting leukemia, and we have developed a bond that goes far beyond a business relationship.

This is the 3rd day of July. Rorie looks wonderful. I expect her to look pale and stressed, but she has a radiance about her. She's suddenly lost six pounds, but she's glad because it's the six pounds we all want to lose. I run into Dr. Minor Vernon, Jessica's pediatrician, who has just heard about Rorie. On the way to lunch, I see Debbie Liipfert, a nurse who directs a program for new mothers. She tells me she would have never suspected anything was going on based on my outward appearance. I guess my exterior isn't betraying me. Debbie becomes one of my closest buddies and gives Rorie and me constant encouragement and words of comfort. A few minutes later I see one of Rorie's nurse friends who tells me to call if I ever need help. I hear from Denny, a nurse and neighbor who even offers to cut the grass. Another doctor friend calls the office and leaves a message that he heard about Rorie and sends his prayers. Dr. Walt Treadwell, our chief of family medicine, comes by my office and is very upset to hear about Rorie. He continues to ask about her frequently. The word has really permeated the Medical Center. I cherish these caring people.

I go to the courthouse because I want to look at a plat book and see the relationship of the lot we want to the main thoroughfare. I run into the chairman of the county commission, and he asks, "Doc, how's your pretty wife?" I hold my breath a moment and say, "Larry, haven't you heard about Rorie? She has breast cancer." I feel like an actor and am just saying my lines. The story is fiction. I can't possibly be standing in the courthouse talking about my wife with breast cancer. On the way out, I see Judge Bill Self, our probate judge, who wants an update. This is the day I encounter the most people wanting to help and asking about Rorie. It is also the day we receive the most mail—nine cards and letters.

At a weekly Sertoma Club meeting, a friend, Robert Oplinger, comes up to me and shakes my hand. He asks about Rorie, and I reply that she's just fine. He says he's glad to know that but then asks, "How are *you* doing?" It reminds me that Rorie and I are a team. We're really going through this together. I don't have her cancer, but it hurts both of us in different and similar ways. I arrive home feeling sorry for myself and a bit down.

On top of the stack of mail is a card from Tim Bagwell. He has left a lifelong impact on me as my minister. I was devastated when he and Susan were transferred. Tim is the rarest of rare human beings who has a wit and charm about him that is unforgettable. His note says simply: "I think of you often. I pray for you frequently. May you feel God's strength." Knowing the journey that Tim and Susan have had through breast cancer, I know he doesn't have to say anything more. I will be forever grateful for this short note that comes at just the right time. Rorie comments that she wishes she could see Tim, if only for a few minutes, because she thinks he can look through her eyes and see her soul.

The 4th of July is a pleasant day with low humidity. Last year we were all in Panama City, and Brooke and I went deep sea fishing looking forward to a fun-filled father and son outing. It was a rough day, and I got deathly seasick and threw up nine times. I didn't think a human being could be that sick and survive. That must be how sick some people can be from chemotherapy. It is indescribable. I am so thankful Rorie hasn't had that kind of reaction.

The first of Rorie's wigs arrives over the weekend. Our kitty, Puss, doesn't like this intruder, but I think it looks just like Rorie's hair without any trace of the gray she dislikes. Brooke tries it on, and well, enough said, then Jessica puts it on and looks just like Rorie. It is remarkable to see how much Jessica looks like her mother if the hair is the same. Rorie finally tries it on. I love it. She hates it. It makes her look like a winner at the Country Music Awards. She doesn't see the humor. I think it takes off about ten years, but Rorie doesn't believe me. I know there will be many more wigs on the way and decide to give each one its own unique name and personality. This one begs to be named Winnie. Rorie is fascinated with her wig catalogs. I know she anticipates having no hair and wants to look as good as she can. She likes lots of shoes, and now she apparently wants lots of wigs from blonde to brunette, short to long, straight to curly.

Church is inspiring again. Hugh preaches about how important it is to have a song in our heart. He tells a true story about a little three-year-old boy who would sing to his baby sister while his mother was pregnant. When the baby was born, there were serious problems, and she was placed in a neonatal intensive care unit. After a while, it looked as though she might die. The doctor allowed the little boy to go into the unit with his mother to sing one last time. He went up to the bassinet and began singing the song he had sung so many times before.

You are my sunshine, my only sunshine,
You make me happy when skies are gray.
You'll never know dear how much I love you,
Please don't take my sunshine away.

After the little boy sang his song, his baby sister improved and soon went home. Rorie is my sunshine, and cancer isn't going to take her away. I look at her every day and see a song in her heart. Once again Hugh provides a sermon that is exactly what we need to hear.

After church we go see the movie *Independence Day*. In one scene the President's wife dies. This upsets Rorie, and she talks about how she would rewrite that part of the movie. We sing "You Are My Sunshine" all day and cook amberjack on the grill.

We receive a card and letter from Phyllis Rooney in Flagler Beach, Florida. She was my supervisor when I was a special education teacher. Phyllis attended our wedding. She has enclosed a letter from one of her friends who was treated for breast cancer. It includes a list of do's and don'ts for someone taking chemotherapy. Yesterday Hugh talked about our needing a song in our heart. Today Phyllis sends the following message:

If you keep within your heart a green bough—I have heard—
there will come one day to stay, a singing bird.

Rorie's collection of cards and letters is impressive.

If the oncology nurse is right, Rorie will lose her hair any day. When I think rationally, I know it will be temporary, and her hair will come back—maybe better than before. But emotionally, I dread the day and selfishly think about my reaction. So far, breast cancer hasn't been as difficult as we thought it would be, but I fear we are in for a rude awakening.

Winnie the wig rode to work with Rorie today on the back seat of the car. Rorie will take it to a hairdresser and see if she can do something about the country and western look. She comes home frustrated because she still doesn't think it looks right. She doesn't want to go to work one day with almost no hair and then come back looking like she is in the Grand Old Opry. Time for bed. Rorie sits on the side of the bed with me and starts to pull long strands of hair out. "It's starting," she sobs. "I was hoping maybe this wouldn't happen." We hug each other and cry. It is precisely two weeks after her first treatment, just like the nurse said. I have been trying to make the wig issue something to laugh about, but tonight I don't have much of a sense of humor. This has to be terribly hurtful and almost unbearable for Rorie. She always takes such pride in her appearance. She won't even go to Kroger if she doesn't look just right.

She has her hair cut real short into what I call a Peter Pan hairdo, and she is buying more wigs by the day. Rorie has an extraordinary resiliency about her. She starts wearing her wigs around the house with a positive attitude that she might as well have fun. At work, she has her Peter Pan look and has not yet worn a wig. Three people make comments. In the cafeteria, one lady asks, "What have you gone and done to your hair?" Another asks, "Why in the world did you cut all that pretty hair off?" Rorie jokes that she's having hot flashes in this July weather and wants a cooler hairdo. A young man who works on her floor comments, "You should have never cut your hair." It's all I can do to keep from grabbing these people and yelling at them that she cut her hair because she has cancer! Rorie has such remarkable courage and patience to be able to handle these kind of remarks. I am frankly stunned by how insensitive some people can be.

On the other hand, we are encountering people full of God's spirit who I believe are already on the heavenly road to becoming an angel. One such angel is June O'Neal, a member of our church, who quietly leaves cookies and cherry pie and other goodies on our backdoor step early in the morning while we're still asleep. Our friends keep calling and sending cards that warm our hearts. For every insensitive person, there are a hundred more who just want to help.

Rorie's wigs arrive. We name the sexy blonde one Candy; the fluffy brown one, Madge, the country club gal; the dark one, Veronica, the sophisticate; and the long brown one, Hillary. One night before Rorie wears her wig to work for the first time, we need a couple of things from the store, so she decides it is time for a trial run. "Who is the most nervous, you or me?" she asks as she gets out of the car and walks into the store. We don't see anyone we know, and there are no odd looks.

All of Rorie's hair finally comes out. There is hair everywhere, on the pillow, the bed, the carpet, and the bathroom floor. I vacuum and sweep, and that is that. When we go to the second chemotherapy session, Rorie has on one of her wigs. Another patient says, "Look, she hasn't lost her hair at all." Rorie gets compliments from people who don't realize she is wearing a wig. One day at Kroger in the vegetable section, a lady wants to know who does her hair because it's just the cut she's been looking for.

The third treatment proves to be the last—at least for now. Each time we go, we meet new friends who share the same fears and anxieties and hope. Cancer is the great equalizer. There is no sense of status when people sit together and receive chemotherapy. There is only a sense of understanding and unspoken faith. Listening to these people, I know that I am not immune from cancer, and one day Rorie may have to sit and hold my hand as I go through treatment. I am learning from her example of courage and faith. In simpler times, we would be getting ready for football season. But now our attention is on surgery and what lies beyond.

SURGERY
Eliminating the Adversary

"When we are in a situation where Jesus is all we have, we soon discover he is all we really need."

—Gigi Graham Tchividjia

Like most little girls, I couldn't wait to grow up. I was anxious to start wearing a bra and shave my legs and leave childhood behind. When I reached puberty and my breasts started developing, I enjoyed my transition into womanhood and looked forward to getting married, having lots of babies, and living happily ever after with a man who loved me. My breasts were part of my sexuality, and, though it wasn't fashionable to nurse when Brooke was born, I cherished the privilege of nursing Jessica. There are many categories of cancer that steal life away from the young and the old, but because of our society's obsession with the breast, my category of cancer stirs up a special array of emotions.

There are literally just days left until I will lose part of me that has been vital in my relationship with Robert and that has helped me fulfill my role as a mother. Now those same breasts have become my deadliest enemies. They must be eliminated. My faith is with God and with Dr. Dale as he uses all his training and skill to remove the source of the cancer that is invading my body. Soon I will lose my breasts to add to my loss of hair.

Dr. Dale prepares me and Robert to expect about four hours of surgery. He tells us he needs a resident with him, so we ask for Dr. Tim Barron, a third-year surgery resident who has become a good friend. Dr. Dale assures us he will make the arrangements. I again ask for David Littleton to be my anesthetist and for Dr. Vince Skilling to be my anesthesiologist. I ask my friend, Brenda, to be one of the OR nurses, and she arranges her schedule to be there. I am prepared to be in the hospital for three days and then stay home for six weeks.

It is the last Sunday in August. After church a little boy who sits in front of us comes up to me and grabs my hand. A victim of abuse beyond comprehension, he now lives at the Methodist Children's Home and has been attending our church the past year. He has become very special to me. Today he beams as he tells me about his favorite song, "Victory in Jesus." He tells me he learned it several

Sundays ago, and the words brought his memory back. I can only imagine what this sweet little boy has had to repress to survive, but Jesus has given him freedom and protection. My little friend has found victory. This is a moment when God is blessing him and speaking to me at the same time. I am thankful I was drawn to church this morning.

Today I hear from Brenda Murphree, a former neighbor. She lost her husband unexpectedly a few months ago, and, though she has her own pain to work through, she has her Sunday School class praying for me. Brenda wants to be there on the day of surgery. I welcome her offer. I never realized how powerful prayer is until so many people started praying for me. There must be hundreds. The power is lifting me up and giving me strength I could never have created through my own will.

On Monday, Dr. Dale comes around the corner and catches me by surprise. I feel a bit wobbly today from thinking about my surgery, but he gives me some words of encouragement, and I feel better. Robert tells me he has a surprise but will not give me any details. After work, we go to Central City Park and wait by the gazebo. I think, "Gosh, this is weird. What is going on?" It turns out that Pauline Thomas, the wonderful lady who greets people when they enter the Medical Center, has prepared a picnic for us. She and her nephew, Tony, unload their car. We have lasagna, salad, garlic bread, and cherry pie. There's that cherry pie again, my favorite. Pauline greets everyone who enters the Medical Center with a smile. She has been very special to me and asks about my progress every day and also prays for me. Today she takes her time off to plan a picnic just for us. I am very moved by this expression of love.

I know that God is with me and I will survive, but my human frailty takes over occasionally, and I feel a sense of despair. I am sure God understands because Jesus felt every human emotion I feel. That is such a miracle. A devotional I read reminds me to slam the door on despair before it drags me down. I know I have to read this every day between now and the 4th of September.

On Friday before Labor Day, I have an emotional time saying goodbye to my friends when I leave work. This is the last time they will see me before my surgery. I try to think about the first football game of the season against Southern Mississippi tomorrow, which is the debut of our new coach, Jim Donnan. Robert and I bought some gray T-shirts a few weeks ago and had them embroidered with a ferocious bulldawg and personalized with Dr. Dawg and Mrs. Dawg. I'm eager to wear my T-shirt while I still have my own breasts, and I will show off my blonde wig to our tailgate buddies in the Science Library parking lot.

Brooke and Leah come up to Athens to the game. Robert is thrilled to get his special parking spot. We have to leave our driveway at precisely 6:15 A.M. for every home game in order to arrive in time to get that special spot where Dr. Dawg can preside. The leaves have already started to turn for an early fall, and our friends greet us with love and prayers for my surgery on Wednesday. We lose the game but win the day with our Bulldawg friends.

The next three days are much like preparing to go on a trip. There are many things to do. I am remarkably calm. I give my toenails a new paint job because I don't want anyone talking about my feet. I worry a bit about being bald in the operating room and wonder if I will have anything on my head. I clean house, pack a bag of supplies for my hospital stay, and make sure the family can all be together for a barbecue on Labor Day night.

On Tuesday, Robert and I go to the mall and eat at the food court. I am so worried about Robert. He is no poker player. I can read him like a book and see so much turmoil in his face. We both agree that we will be much better in a few days when I get back home. I'm faced with the imminent challenge of choosing clothes that will fit and look good after I lose my breasts. This is not something I have had to deal with before. I can't find anything I like. I am glad the weather will soon turn cool so I can wear bulky tops that will camouflage my flat chest. Hugh leaves an inspiring message on the answering machine and promises he will be there in the morning. My bags are packed, and Elmo is ready to go. Nothing left to do but pray, go to sleep, and hand everything over to God.

My despair is taken away, and I sleep well. Robert and I get up early to be at the Surgery Center at 6:00 A.M. I'm on the schedule for 7:40, which means I am Dr. Dale's first case. After a hug from Nan at the front desk, we go upstairs to the sixth floor and get settled into my room. Brenda is waiting. Soon Hugh comes in with his sweet, loving smile. I have a spectacular view of the sun coming up over Macon and think what a beautiful city we have. Jessica, Brooke, and Leah are with me. I'm given some Valium, which doesn't have much effect, and my friend Kim starts an IV. I exchange my wig for a doubled-up hospital cap and want to make sure nobody sees my bald head. Hugh prays with us. His presence is comforting to me, and I know Robert needs him just as much. Hugh promises to stay until I have to leave for surgery.

Dr. Skilling and David come into the room and treat me like I'm the only patient in the universe. David has come in on his day off to be in the OR with me. Dr. Skilling confesses that he has become much more aware of the trauma of breast cancer. He asks Robert if he wants to go into the OR while I'm given the anesthesia. His extraordinary compassion is evident when he observes that since Robert and I go to sleep together every night, Robert needs to be with me when I go to sleep today.

Several of my cohorts from Outpatient Holding come by to see me. My nurse friend Brenda comes in and reassures me she will be there throughout the entire operation and will call Robert from the OR with periodic updates. Also, she has arranged for a special request I made to have a Yanni CD playing in the OR for good luck. Finally, it's time to go. I tell everyone goodbye, except Robert who has put scrubs on and accompanies me to the OR. On the elevator I see my friend J. P., another one of the terrific nurses I have the privilege to work with.

I'm wheeled into the OR and then am shifted onto the operating table. Brenda has already cranked up the "Yanni Live at the Acropolis" tape. Dr. Dale and Dr. Barron are talking about new houses. David and Dr. Skilling are in the room. I'm glad they're with me. Robert holds my hand. Then, in what seems like a minute or two, I am in the recovery room. I have had a modified radical mastectomy on the right side and a simple mastectomy on the left side. I feel foggy, but I see Robert, Jessica, and Brooke. I have no pain, but I'm thirsty. My nurse is excellent. It's not long before another friend, Earl, is wheeling me up to Room 310.

The kids and Robert love my room, which has a stocked refrigerator and lots of snacks. Robert will spend the night with me. We feel like we're in a fancy hotel room. I feel remarkably well so far and am relieved that I do not have a urinary catheter. However, I have to urinate like crazy following four hours worth of IV fluids. I have one drain coming out of my left side and two on the right. I absolutely must go to the bathroom. This is a real struggle and balancing act. I have to scoot the IV pole along and juggle the drains in my sides, but with my nurse's support, I somehow make it and find what can only be described as blessed relief.

My mouth is dry. I have a craving for a hamburger and fries. Robert sends Brooke to MacDonald's to get me what I want, but I can only take a few bites. Later, I get extremely nauseated and throw up volumes of fluids. After I expel everything in my stomach, I feel much better, but still have no appetite. I am connected to a morphine pump. I don't really need it but think, what the heck, I'll give it a try. I use it twice. During the operation, Brenda wrapped a towel around my bald head to keep me covered and warm, so I don't feel very glamorous when our friend, Ronnie Rowe, comes by. A green towel on the head isn't very stylish.

In the morning I wake up famished. For breakfast I eat eggs, bacon, grits, and biscuits and jelly and drink orange juice and coffee. My IV has infiltrated my neck. There is noticeable puffiness. I had to have my IV stuck in my neck in order to keep my arms free during the mastectomies. When it is removed, the swelling subsides. After a sponge bath I can put my wig back on and search for my lipstick. Ronnie Rowe's wife, Kaye, comes by. Many of my hospital buddies drop in while the room fills up with cards and flowers. Robert surprises me with the most wonderful toy red fire engine that has flashing lights and two different sirens. Our Medical Center chaplains, Reverend Tim Price and Father Bob Gibson, make me feel better with a laugh and a prayer. Hugh came by earlier while I was asleep. Dr. Barron comes by, gives me a reassuring hug, and comments on the Yanni CD in the OR. Robert looks exhausted. I know he didn't sleep well on the couch. I send him home for a shower and a nap. Dr. Dale comes by and says I'm doing well.

On Thursday, I feel good and urge Robert to spend the night at home. He looks so tired. All the nurses on every shift are wonderful. In the morning, Robert arrives with the newspaper and coffee and looks rested and happy. We must wait for Dr. Dale's permission to be discharged but are anxious to go home. At noon, Dr. Dale comes in with a medical student and removes my dressings as Robert watches. I am glad Robert seems to accept my condition, and the drains don't appear to bother him. David, my anesthetist, stops by to check on me and tells me he prays before he puts his patients to sleep. His prayers must work because he is one of the best, deserving the nickname, "The Sand Man." Dr. Skilling comes by, and we have a good talk. Then it's time to load up the cart and head for home. I think life is awfully good today. The sunshine looks brighter, the birds sing more beautifully, and my house looks newer. Puss is glad to see me and curls up on the couch as I get comfortable.

A nurse friend and church member, Susie Slappey, has been calling people to join a food patrol to bring us a week-long procession of dinners. She arrives in the afternoon with the most delicious pot roast we have ever enjoyed along with Waldorf salad and brownies. Methodists find a way to associate food with every significant life event from birth to marriage to sickness and death, so I am very fortunate this day to be a member of Martha Bowman church. We savor this wonderful week of food and no cooking.

Now I have to cope with three drains coming out of my sides. Dr. Dale told me I can have them removed when the fluid is less than 30cc. in each one over a twenty-four-hour period. I want to discard these things and get some breast prostheses so I can go out in public and look as normal as possible. My right arm is extremely stiff, but I know I have to keep it moving. I have to empty each drain as it fills, and I do my best to keep clean with sponge baths. I have to sleep on my back, but hate this since I can't roll over and hug Robert. I am starting to discover my new body and try to keep telling myself this will not be me forever. Dr. Dale had to go far up into my right armpit to make sure he got all the lymph nodes that were invaded. The incision left a deep crease that I pray can be improved through reconstructive surgery. I have an appointment with Dr. Dale on

Tuesday. I will find it challenging to figure out a way to hide these infernal drains while out in public.

At Dr. Dale's office, he takes out two of the three drains. I am surprised at how far inside they went. When he removes the first, I gasp. There is no pain, but it feels like a roto-rooter is being pulled out of my chest. He goes over the pathology report with Robert and me and tells us the left side had no lymph node involvement, but of the fourteen lymph nodes removed on the right, seven had cancer. Mom arrives this afternoon with my sister Debby and her daughter, Alex. It is all I can do to keep from crying when I see my mother. I will return to Dr. Dale's office on Friday to get rid of the last drain. More angels from church bring food. The amount of food we are receiving every day is overwhelming.

A couple of days later Dr. Dale removes the last drain and steristrips covering my incisions. Finally, I feel free. Then he gently scolds me for not moving my right arm enough. I am going to have tightness and should also expect to have lymphedema, which is an accumulation of fluid in the arm causing swelling. This is not good news, but I go home looking forward to the privilege of taking a hot shower for the first time in ten days.

I stay home from church because I haven't gotten any prostheses yet, and I am not going out with a flat chest. Later, a volunteer from Reach for Recovery comes by and gives me a pillowlike prosthesis. I try it out and am thankful to have a semblance of a chest. I know right away I will need something more realistic looking. While we visit in my living room, I learn that she had a double mastectomy and reconstruction using tissue expanders. She shows me her breasts, and they look terrific. She is my age and has a wonderful attitude. I hope I can get by with tissue expanders, too, but doubt it because of the radiation I will have to endure. I've heard that if radiation is included in treatment, expanders will not be a viable option. I think about junior high school when some late bloomers stuff socks in their bras and realize that is what I must look like. Mom goes home today but will come back soon. At least we'll see her for sure when we go to Jacksonville for the Georgia-Florida game.

My drain site on the right side isn't healing up as fast as it should. I treat it with peroxide and neosporin. My chest is extremely tender all the way up to my collarbone. My left armpit aches sometimes, even though no nodes were removed. I can move my right arm much better, and the crease in my armpit has improved. But the back of my right arm is numb, although I feel a burning sensation when I touch it. I am not able to sleep like I want, wrapped around Robert, but have to remain on my back. I want to get comfortable, but can't seem to turn on my side without a pulling sensation in my arm. It's time to return to Dr. Schnell. He tells us he is arranging for radiation treatments, which will be followed by two or three treatments of Taxol—more chemotherapy. The good news is that Taxol will be the end of my treatment.

On Friday night, Robert and I sit on the deck and can hear the football game at Jessica's high school. It is a clear, crisp fall night. The moon is visible through the tall Georgia pines. When it's time for bed, I start to cry when I look down at my chest and back up at my bald head. I don't see the person I know in the mirror, and tonight I am unable to smile. Robert and I have invented a code called big cry and little cry, which means sometimes we have pain from deep down in our souls and other times we just need to shed a tear or two and then we're okay. Because Robert is here to hold me close, tonight is only a little cry.

From Robert. . .

For the past few years I have made it a habit of providing the altar flowers at church on the Sunday closest to our wedding anniversary. I write my name on the flower calendar early in the year so I can reserve the Sunday I want. When I wrote my name on the calendar last January, I would have never believed what our life would be like when that special Sunday arrived. I bought the flowers this Sunday, but we stayed home.

On Monday, Debby and Alex leave, but Mary stays behind. June O'Neal leaves a cake topped with cherries. Rorie is a little teary at lunch and says she hates the wig she's wearing today, which I think makes her look like Elizabeth Dole. I have written the first chapter of what I hope will become a book and send it to Tim and Susan Bagwell. I want their reaction because they have so much insight into what I'm trying to communicate. After Rorie and I return home, I go into the bathroom and see the wig in the trash can. I yell to Rorie downstairs that somebody must have broken in and left us some roadkill.

On Tuesday, I decide to act on an idea I've had for a surprise for a long time. I want to get a picture of some firemen and have it enlarged and have all the guys sign it for Rorie. I go by the fire station near the Medical Center and meet Lt. Dewey Davis and tell him my wife has breast cancer and loves firemen and ask if I can take their picture. He is excited about helping me. The firefighters pull the fire engines outside, and I get a great picture of eleven firemen. I'll see them later when I get the picture enlarged.

Jessica is invited to the Optimist Club to talk about her experience as Bibb County Junior Miss. She invites Mary and me, and we attend the breakfast meeting. I am so proud of her and am caught a little off guard by how mature she has become. A former neighbor who is a member of the club hears about Rorie, and he gives me a warm hug. Later in the day Rorie tells me that when she went out to the mailbox to get the newspaper, she looked up into the clear morning sky and prayed, "Oh God, you decided not to take my cancer away, but can you at least stop it from spreading and let me help somebody?" That afternoon, she got a call at work to please come talk to a young girl recently diagnosed with breast cancer and facing chemotherapy.

On Sunday, Rorie wears her Candy wig to church. Several people we know well don't recognize her. Hugh loves it and calls Rorie his blonde girlfriend. Rorie gets a great deal of strength from Hugh. On Monday, I hear about the idea of a Breast Center at the hospital. Rorie is interested in helping out. Already she is becoming a counselor of sorts, and people are seeking her out for advice. Tonight Rorie comes to bed and is unusually quiet. I know she is tormented, so I force the issue. She has been downstairs telling Mary goodbye since she will be leaving for Jacksonville in the morning. Rorie cries and cries. When I demand that she tell me what's wrong, she replies, "I can't say it." I keep pushing, and she says, "I can't say it" at least three times. I have never seen her act like this. Rorie looks so tired. I hug her and ask again. She starts to weep and says, "This may be the last time I see my mother." I am terribly upset and ask why. She sobs, "Because I might die."

Rorie's words devastate me because this is the first time she has ever expressed her feelings that death is a possibility. She is always so upbeat and positive, but I know she has been deeply worried and has had thoughts about death tearing her away from her family. I realize how frightening it is for Rorie to think of leaving her children without a mother and me without a wife. After a few moments, she tells me in a soft voice, "The next time Mom sees me I won't have any breasts." She expresses grief about losing part of her identity. I know she has to get it out of her system. Her mother has visited us many times, but this time her leaving has made the goodbye especially painful.

I feel unbearably stressed and depressed. I want to run away from myself and be somebody else, if only for a day. I've gained some weight because of my depression, then I get depressed because I've gained weight. I get caught in so many vicious circles. No matter what I do, I can't seem to relax. Rorie sees the worry in my face and keeps asking me if I'm okay. I always answer, "I'm fine, I'm fine." Dear God, I know you're there, and I know you love me, but why does this have to hurt so much?

There are only hours left before Rorie will have her mastectomies. We go to the mall, and Rorie has a confident aura of peace about her. I want her sense of peace and her amazing faith. I wonder if I'm doing something to keep God away. Have I closed my heart up to the point where I can't hear God speaking to me? We get a remarkable message from Hugh on our answer machine that gives us both some extra strength. He is our minister and friend, and he is such an anchor during this horrible time in our life. Maybe God is sending Hugh as His messenger. Our Gator friend, Mary Kay, calls from Jacksonville. Rorie's dear nurse buddy, Brenda, calls and says she has everything all lined up. Laurie Gerwig, a friend from church who directs a breast health center at a local hospital, comes by and gives Rorie a hug and encouragement.

On this eve of surgery, the night skies light up with an incredible display of flashing heat lightning. It explodes out from the east, and then is answered from the west, turning the darkness into sheets of brilliant light with no thunder. Surely, Smitty has been able to get permission from God to put on another show for us before the big day. Rorie seems to be drawn into the light of this performance. Her thoughts about her Daddy must give her an extra source of courage.

We arrive at the Surgery Center at 6:00 A.M. Rorie goes by to see her buddies in Outpatient Holding before we ride the elevator up to the sixth floor to Room 23. Rorie gets Valium, then an IV, and then some special hose to prevent blood clots. I think maybe I should have some Valium, too. Vince Skilling comes by and talks from the heart about breast cancer and his concerns about all the cases he's seeing. He and his wife, Nancy, become faithful friends and a central source of encouragement. Hugh comes in carrying his infamous red hat that was given to him by the legendary football coach, Erk Russell. No matter the time of year or the color of his suit, Hugh Davis will have his red hat on. I have come to cherish his red hat as something I always want to see coming toward me if I'm in trouble. Hugh prays a wonderful prayer, and I start to feel a little better. Brenda Murphree, our neighbor from years ago, is with us and will stay until she is sure Rorie's surgery is a success and we have everything we need.

To my surprise, Vince asks if I want to go into the OR until they put Rorie to sleep. I say, "Of course," and awkwardly put on the scrubs with Hugh's help. Soon we are rolling Rorie's stretcher down to the surgery suites on the second floor. The OR is a busy place. I am touched by the love and concern I see expressed for Rorie. These people aren't just doing their jobs; they genuinely love her—and it shows. I hold Rorie's hand, and we look at each other for a moment as though we're alone in the world. David starts to administer the anesthesia. Rorie's chatter begins to slow down, she starts to fade away, and then her eyes stop moving as she loses consciousness. I am not used to seeing someone go under anesthesia and am overcome with how all this must look the same as dying. I have this terrifying thought that I've just seen a preview of Rorie dying. I can't see well because of my tears. Vince asks me if I'm going to be all right as he leads me out of the OR. I can't talk, so I just nod. I find my way back to Room 23 and struggle to gain my composure as Brooke asks, "Dad, are you okay?" My son puts his arm around me. I am thankful this strong young man is with me. We receive six calls from the OR during the operation as Brenda assures us everything is going well.

I find myself alone for a few minutes when everyone goes for coffee and some snacks. I stare at the sun that has come up beautifully over Macon. Brooke will bring me my mid-morning Diet Coke, which is a necessity. I sit there quietly with Elmo in my lap. My heart is peaceful. I discover that God must have been waiting for me to be alone to assure me He will never leave me. I am convinced this new day is for my wonderful wife who has filled my life with love and joy. Then God sends Tim Price into the room who tells me he had a prayer session for Rorie this morning. He has been studying angels and believes as I do that some special people are in the process of becoming angels while still here on earth. These people have extraordinary gifts and a radiance everyone can see. I know that I am married to one of those people as I am reminded of a card Rorie received with a verse, part of which goes:

> *There are some special people*
> *Who are so outgoing,*
> *So self-giving,*
> *So un-self-centered,*
> *So full of good humor,*
> *So interested in others,*
> *And so enthusiastic*
> *That when we see them coming,*
> *We go toward them*
> *For they bring us gladness*
> *And our hearts grow merry*
> *And the day grows brighter*
> *And trees seem greener*
> *And birds sing sweeter*
> *And the sky is bluer*
> *And our cares diminish.*

That is the most accurate description of Rorie I have ever encountered. People are indeed drawn toward her because she makes them feel good about themselves. There is a steady stream of visitors when Rorie is transferred to Room 310 post-operatively. Father Bob comes by and says a prayer. Ronnie Rowe answers the telephone when

Jimmy Taylor calls. After two nights, it is time for Rorie to come home.

Each afternoon there is more food arriving from church. The number of cards has slowed down, but at least one still arrives every day. Rorie's hair is growing back. I pray she won't have to have any more chemotherapy and lose it again. The idea of losing it for a second time bothers me more than the first time for some reason. Rorie is healing quickly. I wonder what our sex life will be like over these next many months. It will be different for both of us, yet I am still very attracted to Rorie regardless of what has happened to her physically. If lovemaking is based on love as it should be, there is no need for us to give up normal marital relations.

I can't imagine how Rorie feels to have such an important part of her body gone. With no breasts she looks so different now in her nightgown. I am gradually accepting this more each day, but I'm not ready to look at her completely nude. I know she has to be terribly self-conscious, but the assurance of reconstruction has to give her courage. Still, we are progressing very slowly to the point where she will be comfortable letting me see her. And I need some time, too.

The photograph of the firemen I had enlarged is ready, so I take it to the fire station, but learn they are all gone to a controlled fire for some training. I find the street where they're training and see Lt. Dewey. He gathers the crew around, and they take off their gloves and sign Rorie's picture while we hold it flat on the hood of a car. It's signed with each of their names. Lt. Dewey writes, "Best Wishes to Rorie, Engine #10, Truck #31." Now I will take it and have it prepared with a red mat and black frame. It will be ready in a couple of weeks. Rorie is going to love this. I cannot wait.

The doorbell rings one afternoon. It is a friend of Rorie's. She presents Rorie with four certificates to have the house professionally cleaned plus two cards signed by all the girls in the neighborhood. This is a welcomed, thoughtful, and creative gift. Rorie is told that she gives all of them hope, and, while they don't see her every day, they are watching and praying and cherish her example. Rorie is very touched. This makes me realize how people observe Rorie and me and, though they don't say something every day, wonder how we are coping. Rorie is an inspiration to people she doesn't even know.

At the end of September, we attend our annual cardiology conference at St. Simon's Island. We are with good friends, but we steal away
one evening and have a pizza at a little place called CJ's. It is a popular
spot, and people have to wait to get inside. Rorie is very sensitive to
how other women look, and she gets tearful about not having any
breasts. I tell her that some of the girls in the restaurant may be going
through breast cancer themselves and think she looks good and she is
the lucky one. We never know when we look at other people what
they may be experiencing. Back at our room, it is a beautiful night
with the moon shining over the ocean. Rorie steps out on the balcony.
I leave her alone for a few minutes because I know she needs to think
and probably say a prayer. Then I join her, and we kiss and make love
with the moonlight filling every corner of our room. There will be no
barriers to our intimacy. We can still be close and find each other
exciting.

The next day Rorie is happy and has put on her shopping face.
She and Betty Treadwell decide to go looking for antiques. They have
a great day. Later, a crowd of us go to Blanche's Courtyard for dinner,
and we have a wonderful evening. I want this weekend to go on and
on, but I know that radiation has to begin on Monday. It's time to
move on to still another mode of treatment, even though I find it
difficult to conceive of this ever ending.

RADIATION
Enduring the Reality

"Faith isn't the ability to believe long and far into the misty future. It's simply taking God at His word and taking the next step."

—Joni Erickson Tada

I sometimes hear cancer treatment options referred to as poison, slice, and burn, which of course are cynical ways of looking at chemotherapy, surgery, and radiation. So I've already experienced the poison intended to kill my cancer cells, the slicing to remove the cancer in my breasts and lymph nodes, and now it's time to get burned by radiation. As much as I pray and spend time with God, I cannot help but grow weary through this process to save my life. I will do all that I must, and I will listen to my doctors, but I have to be honest and say that I am being worn down. I have had strange heart palpitations recently, and I am worried.

On Monday morning, I go to the ground floor of the Doctors Building for my appointment with Dr. Drew Cole, my radiologist. His assistants are waiting for me. I am weighed, which is a requirement I always dread. I'm pleased to discover I've lost four pounds. I change into a tiny gown, which keeps falling open. Dr. Cole is detained by another patient's needs and comes into the room about thirty minutes later. He is a very nice young fellow, and I enjoy exchanging some pleasant chitchat with him. He tells me I will have at least thirty-three treatments lasting about five minutes each and occurring each weekday until I am finished. I will have a rest on weekends. There will be a slight sunburn appearance, possible skin irritation, and a very minor possibility of lung damage. He assures me he has never seen that happen, but I think it must happen to somebody if it needs to be mentioned. Also, I could develop low blood platelets, so I will have a complete blood count performed each week to monitor any changes.

I am told that during the last few days of treatment I will get an extra boost of radiation directly on the incision. All the radiation is targeted to my right side, the source of my troubles. I am escorted into another room displaying a huge table and intimidating equipment. I'm carefully placed on this cold, hard table, with my right arm up behind my head and put into sort of a brace. A long series of measurements and calculations are made by Dr. Cole and his nurse. The process involves lights, charts, x-rays, and this strange machine rotating around me. I'm in the room for an hour and a half during which I feel like a big slab of meat. My feelings aren't the doctor's or nurse's fault. They are doing everything they can do to help me. But when they leave the room, I have to fight back tears because I feel like it is a scary movie and I am the star.

Turquoise and red marks are drawn all over my chest like a roadmap, and a huge turquoise mark is placed right on my lower neck that shows over my collar. This is absolutely unacceptable, and it leaves me shaken. I go home and can think of little else than this obvious mark on my neck and what I'm going to do about it. I am a crying mess tonight and have one of my big cries, while poor Robert has the unenviable assignment of making me feel better while he has a terrible cold and feels awful himself. I have to go back to the radiologist tomorrow for more preparation.

My second session lasts only twenty minutes. I am thrilled to have the big turquoise mark replaced with a small tattoo. I see an old friend, Teresa, who was in my Bible study class. She tells me she was devastated when she heard about me. She is a radiation oncology nurse. I am very happy to have such a good contact. The next day I have an appointment with Dr. Dale, who says I'm doing well, and then I return to radiology for still more calculations. I do not enjoy any of this, but I realize how important it is for precision. I know I am getting the best quality care available anywhere.

Robert goes with me for the first treatment. It is scheduled for 11:00 A.M. We plan to meet each day for treatment and then go to lunch together. I am nervous. I sign in. After a short wait, I'm back on that table, in position. Everyone leaves. I am alone. I hear a loud noise. A red light flashes on the wall fifty-two times. The door opens, and one of the techs comes in and repositions the overhead machine. She leaves, the noise is back, and the light flashes fifty-two times again. This happens three times, and then the session is over. I don't feel anything but am glad to return to the waiting room and go to lunch. We come back the next day at the same time. A plastic weighted cover is draped over my chest. I get some kind of boost to the surface tissue that will reoccur every other session. I feel good, and there is no redness on my chest.

Robert arrives home after work with quite a surprise for me. He yells for me to get out of the kitchen before he opens the door. He tells me to close my eyes. Then he presents me with an enormous framed photograph of a gorgeous group of firemen. Each one has signed his name. I am speechless. Robert must have taken a lot of time and effort to do this. It is such a unique and clever idea. He knows how I'm intrigued with firemen and fire engines. This is such a lift to my spirits. Now, where in the world am I going to put this thing? It is a cherished gift, but it's not what you want to put over the mantle.

My third treatment starts to become routine. Robert invites me to lunch at the Green Jacket, and he has the firemen picture with him. He wants to show it to my buddies in Outpatient Holding. They get a hoot out of it and drool over the handsome firemen. On the way to lunch, Robert makes a wrong turn. I realize, oh no, he's headed to the fire station. We arrive, and I want to go in, but I feel kind of embarrassed. Luckily, Lt. Davis is there. I am so happy to meet him and some of his men. They haven't seen the final framed version of the picture, and they are proud and seem touched by what they see and why it was done. I am in heaven in the fire station. These guys are so handsome. I am downright giddy and probably make a fool of myself staring at all the boots, jackets, and helmets. This is a wonderful treat for me.

Robert's sister, Nancy, and her daughter, Laurie, are on the way up from Jacksonville. We clean house like crazy. They have never been to Macon. It is so good to see them. We go to the Whistle Stop Cafe for lunch and have a great visit. They don't seem to be bothered by my wig. They give me love and encouragement. This is a good weekend.

It's back to work on Monday. I resume my radiation sessions. I am starting to see some redness, which looks like a sunburn after the first day at the beach. My heart palpitations are getting worse. I try to ignore them but can't. Robert, Jessica, and I head to Athens for the Tennessee game and stay at the Courtyard Marriott, which has become our headquarters. Jessica wants to go downtown to a coffee shop by herself, and we go around and around on why she can't go. She will be in Athens in September as a freshman, and I want to coach her now on being safe. We have a terrific barbecue in the Science Library parking lot with our Bulldawg friends. It is perfect weather.

We lose the game, but again win the day. I don't tell anyone, but my heart is really worrying me. Maybe the radiation is stressing me, and the fatigue I feel is taking a toll on my heart.

On Tuesday, Brooke calls me and tells me Puss can't stand up and is acting strange. We had a heavy rain a day or two ago, and she disappeared for a day—which has never happened before. Something is seriously wrong. Brooke takes her to the vet and hears that she may have been poisoned. Whatever the reason, she is dangerously anemic, and her kidneys are shutting down. Robert and I are miserable with worry all day. I decide that if my kitty is going to die, she will die at home, so I go by and pick her up from the vet's after work.

When Robert arrives, I have Puss lying on the carpet in the dining room on a blanket. She is cold to the touch. I try to talk to her and give her some iron drops and antibiotics. Robert is terribly upset but tries to be optimistic. When we go to bed, we take her upstairs and lay her on a blanket by the bed. I give her some water. She lets out several unusual breathing sounds and then seems to be alright. We go to bed hoping for a miracle. When I check on her later, she is still alive. About 4:00 A.M. I wake up but cannot bring myself to look at her. I am afraid and wake Robert up. He jumps out of bed and leans down over her and cries, "Rorie, she's dead." We cry and hold on to each other as if a child has died. This was our little pet and friend for more than eight years. We just are not ready for this. It is so quiet and dark. I know Robert is thinking, first the cat, and then you.

Robert puts on his clothes and goes outside in the dark and digs a big grave behind the stack of firewood. Then he comes inside and carries our little kitty downstairs and wraps her up in her white towel that she always slept on. He is almost numb with grief. I hold the flashlight as Robert lays her in the grave and sobs as he covers her with dirt. Then he stacks a small pile of firewood over the spot, and we go back inside. What a sight this would be in the daylight! There I am in my nightgown, totally bald with a flat chest, both of us crying out by the firewood. I grieve all day and worry about Robert. When we come home, he goes straight out to the grave and just stands there. I know there is nothing I can do.

A week has gone by since Puss died. I have gotten rid of the reminders around the house. We miss her, but each day is easier. I am thinking about another pet because I believe it will be good for Robert and me, but he says he doesn't want another animal for a long time.

My chest is itching. I have what can best be described as a heat rash. And I am experiencing what must be hot flashes. I've always joked about women having hot flashes, not understanding what they are like. But these episodes are becoming frequent. My period has stopped, and now I have hot flashes. Have chemotherapy and radiation brought on menopause? I can't be menopausal, at least not until after my high school reunion. Thank God for Gayle Plekowski, a nurse friend who gives me a handheld battery-operated fan to cool me down. This thing is great. Gayle gave me my Elmo doll, and she always comes up with the right gift at the right time. What a friend!

On Friday, Brenda Scherer gives me a guardian angel pin she wore during a rough period in her life. Now she wants me to wear it and then one day give it to someone else in need. She is another one of those angels Robert talks about.

Tonight is Robert's Sertoma Club installation party, which we always attend. Robert has been so active in this civic club for more than twenty years, having been a Gold Honor president a few years ago. But tonight we are very tired and decide that this one time we will not go—everyone will understand. The telephone rings about 8:00 P.M. Pat Meyer wants to know if we're coming and says it's very important to be there. I am exhausted, but Robert hurriedly gets dressed and rushes to the party. As a complete surprise, he is named Sertoman of the Year, the only award he has never received and the one he values the most. Of all nights, I am not there to share this important event with him. I am so sorry.

It's Georgia-Florida time. We went to our first Georgia-Florida game in 1973. The only one we've missed since then was when the Bulldawgs had to go to Gainesville, Florida, in 1994. Though Georgia still leads the series, Florida has been winning every year since Steve Spurrier arrived as coach. The game itself hasn't been as much fun in recent years, but this is a time to go home to Jacksonville and see many friends. This year we stay with Mom one night and then drive to the Marriott Sawgrass for the second night. We discover we've chosen the Gator headquarters, of all places. We go to dinner and sit next to Mel Tillis and have a nice visit with this friendly celebrity. On

Saturday, in the Jaguar Stadium parking lot, I have the worst attack of heart palpitations yet. They make me dizzy and short of breath. I am very fatigued but still go on into the game. I am relieved that the game gets out of hand early and we are able to leave during the third quarter and go back to Sawgrass. I cannot go on any longer with this heart problem and will see Dr. Schnell immediately when we get back to Macon.

Dr. Schnell sees me right away and orders blood work and a chest x-ray and a heart monitor that I will wear through the weekend. My heart flutters get better—probably because I have a monitor. (It's like taking your car to a mechanic because of a funny noise that disappears as soon as the mechanic listens to the engine.) But in church I have a very frightening attack and think I am going to pass out. This scares my family and me, but the monitor never detects anything serious.

Dr. Schnell decides I should see a cardiologist. I am referred to Dr. John Hawkins, a very likable, easygoing man. I have an echocardiogram that shows healthy valves. My EKG is also normal. Dr. Hawkins thinks my palpitations are the result of a combination of chemotherapy, radiation, fatigue, and stress. He prescribes Tenormin, which helps my heart beat more regularly, and I experience immediate improvement.

I continue to go to the radiologist each weekday, and Robert always goes with me. My skin looks like a severe sunburn. I am concerned, but am assured it will clear up. I see the same people each day in the waiting room who are undergoing treatment like me. We have become friendly. Some people want to visit, but others never look up. I know they are going through a trying time, and maybe some don't have the support I am blessed with. As my treatment comes to an end, I have to face more chemotherapy. My hair is just now getting back to the point where I can get by without a wig. But I won't bother, because I know my hair will be gone again in a few weeks.

From Robert. . .

The cat dies, and we close on our building lot on Somersby Lane. Isn't it curious how life's events can contrast so in one day? This morning before daylight I am digging a grave for my little friend that was our pet for as long as we have lived in our house. She showed up the day we moved in, and the pretty kitten that appeared to be about eight weeks old never left. We tried to give her away but failed, and our commitment to her was so fragile we didn't even bother to come up with a proper name. It was simply, "Puss." But she wanted to stay with us, and she gave all of us years of pleasure. Since Puss was one of God's little creatures, before I go back into the house to get her, I say a prayer and express thanks for the opportunity to have her as a member of the family. Everyone with a pet eventually suffers a loss, but Puss couldn't have chosen a worse time to get sick and die.

It is very difficult going to work today, but no one knows how I'm grieving. The end of the day brings a certain amount of joy as we are able to buy the lot we have been dreaming about. If all goes well, we can start building in April or May. I am so glad. This will give Rorie much to think about as she starts collecting magazines with pictures of kitchens and house furnishings. There will be life after cancer, and we will have a new home.

When Georgia-Florida time arrives, I am anxious to go to Jacksonville and see my friends from the Florida Medical Association. We have lunch on Friday at Jacksonville Landing with Ed Hagan and our Gator friends, Mary Kay and Joey. Everyone is thrilled to see Rorie looking so well, and her blonde wig is a big hit. Rorie has developed an appreciation for blonde jokes and, when she makes a mistake, she quickly blames it on her blondeness. The night before, Jessica and I go to see my old high school sweetheart, Brenda North, and her pretty daughter, Natalie. This is a wonderful treat to see them, and our daughters seem to like each other. Brenda and I dated all the way through high school, and though our plans to marry never materialized, we've been friends over the years. This is a good weekend to do some catching up. But we lose the football game, as usual, and Rorie has more heart flutters that worry me.

November 10 arrives. It is Rorie's birthday. We are asked to substitute teach at church in the Sonshine Class for children with special needs. No children show up, so we go on to the 11:00 A.M. worship service. We hear that two young mothers in our church have died from cancer. They die; Rorie lives. Why are we being spared? Hugh preaches that when the going is good, watch out. He tells us that the Sea of Galilee is alive because it gives and receives, while the Dead Sea is dead because it only receives. So no matter how we are down-trodden, we need to help others somehow.

Thanksgiving comes. It is the most important Thanksgiving we have ever celebrated. The house if full, and Rorie's spirit is beaming. She asks me to say the blessing, but I am unable to talk. We have so much to be thankful for that my emotions get the best of me, so Rorie thanks God for His love and for bringing us so far. There is a long way to go still, but I know Rorie is going to make it to the finish.

The season between Thanksgiving and Christmas always causes me to pause and do a fair amount of reflecting. On the first Sunday in December, we stay home from church. While reading the paper, I listen to the television preacher talk about Barabbas, the robber. He reminds us that when the people had a clear choice between freeing Jesus or Barabbas, they chose the robber. And don't we still do it today? Rather than choose Jesus, we choose what will rob us, what will take what is valuable in our lives. I know that much of my stress and depression is my choice. I choose these feelings that rob me of my physical and emotional strength. My prayer for this season is to come to terms with Rorie's cancer and to start investing my energy toward our future.

Rorie's radiation treatment finally comes to an end. When we started, I began a countdown beginning with 33. It is a joy to say goodbye to the nice people in the radiology office. During those days sitting in the waiting room I noticed an elderly couple who came in each day. The tall old gentleman would sit patiently while his wife received her treatment. He would sometimes talk to people he seemed to recognize. I developed a great appreciation for his wisdom and intelligence. This dignified old man knew God personally and possessed a wealth of information about how to live a good life. We would nod and wave to each other as Rorie and I left every day, but I never actually sat down next to him and engaged in a conversation. I was always thinking about myself and absorbed with my troubles, and I was in a hurry to leave. I would learn a few weeks later in Dr. Schnell's office that this interesting old man died. I never knew his name, but I felt a great loss, and I was ashamed that I didn't take advantage of the opportunity to talk with him. Like the people who chose Barabbas, I chose my troubles instead of a valuable chance to learn something from a very wise man.

CHEMOTHERAPY
Closing the Door

"My God is changeless in His love for me, and He will come and help me."

—Psalm 59:10 LB

From Rorie...

I have lost my hair, had my breasts removed, and now I have a burned chest. I really do not want to go through any more chemotherapy. No matter what Dr. Schnell and Robert say I must do, I just don't want any more. Isn't there some way to determine that all the cancer cells are gone, and if so, let me go and have my breasts reconstructed?

Robert always finds a football analogy, so he says we're first and goal with one minute remaining to win the national championship. And if I don't have this last series of chemotherapy, it will be like fumbling and turning the ball over to the opponent. My lack of football knowledge prevents me from fully appreciating his point, but I suppose we have to give my cancer a final kick in the teeth while it's down. How's that for an analogy?

Dr. Schnell tells me I will start Taxol treatment in about a week. This will involve a three-hour infusion every three weeks for four sessions. Each session will be preceded by a dose of Decadron to reduce the risk of an allergic reaction. Side effects can include mild to severe aching joints, peripheral neuropathy, and, of course, absolute hair loss. I have known about this added chemotherapy for a long time, but listening to Dr. Schnell makes me very sad. I have been concerned about weight gain due to the steroids, but I am assured that is not a problem. Maybe the three-hour infusion time scares me since it's twice as long as my first treatments. Maybe I'm just tired of all this powerful stuff being put into my body. But I trust Dr. Schnell with my life—which is exactly what I'm doing.

Work proves to be a successful day. My friend Ruthie and I help one of our ophthalmologists with his eye patients. We do a great job and get complimented. Later in the week Robert and I travel to Atlanta for the American Medical Association interim meeting. I'm so happy to go since we had to miss the annual meeting last June. We see our friend Dr. Yank Coble who has recently lost his wife, Ohlyne, to cancer. It is difficult to know what to say. He looks at me and gives me an understanding hug, telling me I look wonderful. We see our close friend, Bob Seligson, and we laugh and joke around. I feel good. Robert and I stay in the same hotel as the Southeastern Conference Championship headquarters. We see lots of SEC football coaches. We're glad to get to talk with Vince Dooley, and Robert is thrilled to meet Archie Manning, although I don't have any idea who he is. It is so liberating to go around Atlanta where no one knows me or knows about my cancer.

I am reading everything I can about Taxol. Robert printed some articles off the Internet. I am learning that knowledge really is power. I am prepared for treatment more than any time so far, and I want to get it over with. Robert must go to a conference in New Orleans. This will be the first time I have gone to chemotherapy without him. While he's gone, I hope to feel well enough to go to the Surgery Center Christmas party at the new Georgia Music Hall of Fame. Jessica will take me to work and come get me after the session so I won't be concerned with driving.

Though we are all focused on my problems, life has been going on as busy as ever. Jessica has been in the Holiday Spectacular dancing all over the stage, and Robert has been invited to Asheville, North Carolina, to interview for a position as executive director of the Mountain Area Health Education Center. He's perfectly qualified for the job, but in my heart I do not want to leave all the friendships we've developed over the years in Macon. And I want to build our dream house on Somersby Lane. I will go with him and support what-ever decision he makes, but my heart is not in North Carolina.

Robert has left for New Orleans. I miss him. I am feeling a little panic-stricken today and have a long talk with Jesus. I call out to him, and he rescues me. I feel like he walks along with me and touches me. That is the mental image I have, and it gives me comfort. Robert has prepared a Christmas letter to go out to friends letting them know how I'm doing. He hates these things because people often do so much bragging, but he can't stand the idea of writing a personal note over and over. Our friends will understand. I am so anxious to arrive at the day when I don't have to discuss cancer anymore.

This is Friday the 13th, the day I will begin my treatment with Taxol. Brooke calls and tells me he has gotten a job with the Medical

Center. We are thankful and overjoyed. This good news before my session helps my attitude. I arrive at 1:50 P.M. and am not finished until 7:00. I am given Benadryl and Decadron before the Taxol. The infusion takes almost four and a half hours, but I feel fine other than a little racing heartbeat. I sense that Jesus is with me as I sit here.

On Sunday, I can barely move. I feel like I've been hit by a truck. Every bone in my body aches, but I manage to go to church with Brooke and Leah. The youth choir sings some Christmas songs, which helps my attitude. Our friend Jill is sitting behind me. She is on oxygen. I am terribly worried about her, but I can see the strength of her spirit in her smile. On Monday, I am in pain but go to work. On Tuesday, I can barely walk. My feet are killing me, but my condition improves throughout the day. It is abundantly evident that this round of chemotherapy will not be as easy as the first. It's as though they've saved the best for last.

Christmas is here, and Robert has given me an adorable female Yorkie puppy. He said he never wanted another pet when Puss died, but that firm position lasted exactly two months. Robert's mother, Annie Laurie, came from the Wiltshire clan, so this is a perfect name for our new addition. But this puppy's personality isn't quite so regal, so we settle on a nickname, "Peanut." On Christmas Eve we go to church and then come home for a big pot of Minnesota wild rice soup. We have a roaring fire in the fireplace. Our huge tree will be the last one we have in this house. Robert is sitting quietly in his grandmother's rocking chair in front of the tree. I see that his mind is a thousand miles away. He is concerned about me and Jill, and he is having a worrisome time tonight.

On Christmas Day, I have a tingling in my toes and fingertips as the peripheral neuropathy kicks in just like Dr. Schnell warned me. Mom, Debby, and Alex are on the way from Jacksonville. I experience some flu-like symptoms but continue to go to work. I notice that I am much more fatigued than with the first round of chemotherapy. What little hair I have is falling out. I will shave my head right away and be done with it. I am losing all the hair on my body—all of it. I see my eyebrows and eyelashes disappearing and feel like I will soon have to draw my face on every morning.

New Years Eve arrives, and we want so much to put 1996 behind us. Robert and I are thrilled to have seen Tim and Susan Bagwell yesterday at the Medical Center while Tim's father had some surgery. Susan looks wonderful, and I love her hair. She inspires me. Our friends, the Sandefurs, invite us to a party. It is good to get out of the house. When we see our friends, the guys are outside in the backyard, and the gals are in the den. We hug everybody, and I get compliments on my wig. Several friends haven't seen me since my diagnosis, and I detect some quick glances at my chest. This is to be expected. I would do the same. Is that Rorie in there? Has she had reconstruction yet? I know there are some questions that are never asked. Robert usually is so full of information, he provides the answers before I get the questions. This is an important evening for us. We are able to just sit back and relax with friends we love. We laugh, sing, dance, blow horns, and wear silly hats. I am once again thankful.

After the long holiday weekend, I find myself sitting in a motel room in Asheville. Robert is being interviewed Sunday afternoon and evening and all day Monday. We have toured the impressive Biltmore House, so now I am ready to go home. I thought I would be unable to go because of another chemotherapy session, but I am late getting my prescription for Decadron, so treatment is postponed. Robert thought he might have to travel alone, and he was not happy. But we are able to go together and enjoy the beautiful ride up through the mountains, stopping to eat at the famous Dillard House just before leaving Georgia. I have devoted years to developing friends in Macon and don't want to start over. I love my church and my job. And what about Brooke and Jessica? The Sertoma Club is vitally important to Robert, and there is no club in Asheville. And of course, Robert is carefully measuring the distance in time and miles to his parking spot in Athens. There proves to be no compelling reason to move to North Carolina. We decide that our life should remain in Macon and that we are destined to build our new house on Somersby Lane. Thank God.

Back home, Jessica tells us that Jill has died. I think immediately of our incredible moment together in the healing service. My soul feels joy in her victory in Jesus. I grieve for Wally, but know that everyone who knows and loves Jill will have celebration in their hearts.

Her cancer is finally defeated, and she is surrounded by a love beyond anything I can imagine.

I have another treatment. There is an interesting new side effect. As the infusion ends, I see bubbles floating around in front of my eyes. Robert naturally makes a Lawrence Welk joke. I experience aching joints again, and my feet simply hurt. I have a bout of diarrhea and have to urinate frequently. I want to stop my treatment. I am convinced I've had enough and don't need the last two infusions. My hot flashes seem more frequent, and I have uncontrollable mood swings. I am so tired of feeling this way.

Robert takes another trip to New Orleans. I fly there alone to join him. It is the week before Mardi Gras, but the craziness has already begun. We have a Hurricane drink at Pat O'Brien's and dinner at Paschal Manale's. The next morning I am very sick, and Robert teases me that a Hurricane must be worse than chemotherapy. We take a buggy ride into the French Quarter, but get turned back because the crowd is so dense and unruly. It is frightening for the mule and us until we get away from all the rowdy party goers. We decide that we will never go to Mardi Gras if this is a typical preview of what will happen next week.

It's true that I do not want any more chemotherapy, but I am pressured by my family. They love me and don't want me to be miserable, but they want me to get well, and that requires more chemicals in my veins. I have another treatment. Mom is here with me. I am so glad she's visiting, but I hate the idea of her being in a situation to watch her daughter take chemotherapy. My insides are irritated—mucositis it's called—and I have an incessantly runny nose. I ache all over, and now my face is starting to break out. On top of everything else, my feet itch as though I've been standing in an ant bed. It is horrible. Dr. Schnell isn't sure how to stop the itching, but I find that soaking my feet in ice cold water is very effective.

Valentine's Day greets me with a dozen red roses from Robert. I have an appointment with Dr. Schnell, and my last treatment is tomorrow. I enjoy my visit with Dr. Schnell. We talk about New Orleans, and he tells me he will see me in a month and then every six months. He says I will not have to take any more medicine after tomorrow. It takes a moment for this to completely sink in, even though he told me the same thing many weeks ago. No more chemotherapy. No more chemotherapy. Those are beautiful words. When I arrive home, I see a lucky lady bug inside the kitchen window. Brooke is moving into his first apartment and is doing well on his new job. Jessica has been named a National Merit Scholar finalist. There is good news everywhere in my life, and I thank God who has never failed me.

I will always remember Thursday, February 27, 1997. It is a rainy day. Robert is with me. He complains about being cold, but I am miserably hot. This is the first time there has ever been a problem locating a vein for my IV. My nurse, Lynn, who got me started on chemotherapy in the beginning many months ago, is with me and finds a vein. She is very good at infusion. We have become friends, as I have with all the nurses in Dr. Schnell's office. I have been in high spirits all day, but now I feel tired. Soon my session is over. I am given a terrific baseball cap as a graduation present. Robert and I hug everyone and, though I am ecstatic, it is a little sad saying goodbye to Lynn, Mary, and Wanda who have shown so much concern and love over the months. I know they make friends with patients who sometimes die. Their job has to be heartbreaking at times. I will see Dr. Dale tomorrow and then will be ready for reconstruction.

Dr. Dale examines me and says I have minimal deformity and can have any type of reconstruction I want. I have visions of walking down the beach in a few months with a tiny waist and beautiful, perfectly-shaped breasts. I have become accustomed to the side effects of chemotherapy, but this last treatment clobbers me. I feel dizzy with some vision problems, and my itchy feet are driving me crazy. It is almost indescribable.

A friend at the hospital approaches me today. She has had a troublesome mammogram and wants to talk. Her gynecologist suggests she get checked again in six months. Her mother had breast cancer. I tell her my story about delaying and delaying and my denial. I beg her to see Dr. Dale immediately. I don't want anyone to go through what Robert and I have endured.

I am entering an exciting period of life now. I am going to build a house with Robert and have my body rebuilt at the same time. I say a prayer and make an appointment with Dr. Powell. The cherry blossoms are popping out in the front yard. Easter is in the air. I am getting a second chance on life. I will savor and cherish every moment. Resurrection has a special meaning for me this year.

From Robert . . .

It is the first Friday in December. I have decided to take the day off and get some peace and quiet while Rorie and Brooke are at work and Jessica is at school. Rorie starts another round of chemotherapy next week. The pretty hair that has tried to come back will be a goner. It is a beautiful fall morning. I take Jessica's portable CD player and go for a walk listening to a Celine Dion CD. I really like the song she sings, "Call the Man, He's Needed Here." It reminds me that I'm needed and my family loves me. I sometimes think I've been a better husband than a father, but I guess only Brooke and Jessica can be the judges of that.

After several times around the half mile or so route through my neighborhood, I spot a piece of paper lying on the ground by our empty garbage can. Friday is garbage day, so I think this is just some leftover trash. As I lean over to pick it up, I recognize that it's a note I left to Jessica from Santa years before when she was a little girl. Rorie had been cleaning out some closets, and this note found its way into the trash. My routine as Santa was to take advantage of the cookies and milk Jessica would leave. (I would always make sure there were some crumbs on the dish as evidence that Old St. Nick had actually made it down the chimney.) In my purposely large print I wrote,

Dear Jessica,

So many nice things you left me this year. You are an artist. My reindeer were tired and hungry until we stopped at your house. I'll be back!

Love, Santa

I don't know why that one piece of paper fell to the ground and avoided the garbage collector. But I pick it up, fold it, and place it in my diary. I don't think I'm ready to let it go. I think I'll keep it a while.

Christmas and New Years bring with them special emotions as I feel blessed that Rorie has done so well. Yet I am stressed and disheartened. Her hair was growing, and she appeared so strong and healthy. Now, as I look at Rorie asleep with the covers pulled up under her chin, she looks more vulnerable than ever. I have never seen a human being with so little hair. I think the lack of eyelashes bothers me the most. Rorie has such spirit, but I feel like we're going backwards at times. I talk to Jesus and am at peace for a while, then I have to go back and talk with him again. I have to keep going back to the well, so to speak, and quench my thirst for the strength Jesus can give me. I have felt alone frequently, but I have the assurance that Jesus knows exactly how I feel and what I think. Though my sins are many and my faith is weak, Jesus stays with me.

It is very painful when Jill dies. Hugh conducts the service. Tim and Susan are sitting in front of us. I'm not sure, but this may be the first time they have been back to Martha Bowman church since being transferred to Albany. Jill's service is beautiful, and we can feel the love pouring out for her and Wally and their family. There are lots of tears—and laughter. There is a sense of celebration for the way Jill fulfilled her many roles in life. As we are leaving and speaking to Wally, he tells us how much Jill would talk about Rorie and pray for her. We are forever thankful for the love we feel from these two friends.

Rorie and I finally go to her last chemotherapy treatment. There are two very nice ladies sitting across from us. One of them is here for chemotherapy. Her sweet smile and demeanor remind me of my mother. The other lady is her friend who has come along for company. They seem to be impressed with Rorie's attitude and want to talk with us. We mention that we are writing a book. They are very intrigued, so I get their names and addresses and send them a copy of the first chapter. When it's time to leave, there is a mixture of joy and bittersweet emotions since we have become so close to the nurses. It has been raining most of the day, but on the road in the direction of our house just before we arrive home, the threatening dark clouds open up, and beautiful rays of sunlight come shining through. Rorie turns to me and says, "There's my silver lining," and I believe her with all my heart.

In a few days, both of the ladies who were in Dr. Schnell's office write to us and tell us they were inspired and uplifted by the book chapter I sent them. Rorie and I get great satisfaction knowing that these ladies whom we had just met appreciate our message. A few days later, Rorie and I receive word that our book proposal has been accepted. We know our prayers are being answered. This begins a series of events we never anticipated, but we believe God must be orchestrating them. We find ourselves being able to tell our story so that in some small way we might be able to help others facing the same challenging circumstances.

RECONSTRUCTION
Licking Honey off a Thorn

"She has achieved success who has lived well, laughed often, and loved much."

—Bessie Anderson Stanley

From Rorie. . .

Chemotherapy is over for the second time. I am ready to focus on nothing but reconstructive surgery. Dear God, am I ever ready! I have been through many trials and want to focus all my energies on myself and my family. But I encounter Dr. Dale, who asks me if I will serve as a team captain for the American Cancer Society Relay for Life, which is scheduled around the time I will have surgery. I don't think of myself as an organizer, and I've never been involved in this project. Robert and his Sertoma Club have participated a couple of years. I remember Robert coming home all sweaty and proud of himself after running for an hour on a Saturday morning to help raise money for cancer research. He would walk in with a T-shirt and be smug all day for having done such a good deed. I thought it was a good cause but never dreamed it would have any relevance to me.

At about the same time, Robert tells me he has been asked to speak to the church about this event and encourage everyone to form teams. There are many others in the church who have been affected by cancer, and so we know we can only answer yes. Robert speaks at our church Wednesday night supper and becomes very emotional as he tells everyone I am finished with chemotherapy and there will be no more. This is vitally important to say to those assembled because the church has been our rock through this long battle. Later he wears his Relay for Life T-shirt and speaks to all three services on Sunday morning. The church responds with an outpouring of love, and teams begin to come together. At the Medical Center, the Relay for Life becomes a major focus, and at least thirty-four teams register for the event.

In April, our local CBS affiliate, Channel 13, begins planning for a year-long series to encourage women to get a mammogram. The station contacts Focal Pointe Women, a service of the Medical Center, and asks who will be good subjects to interview. Our names are suggested. In about a week, Robert and I are interviewed in our living room by Tina Hicks, one of the news anchors. When Tina and her cameraman arrive, they rearrange our furniture, moving our easy chairs in front of the fireplace so the mantle is in the background. Since we're going to be on TV, I think how lucky we are to have some new furniture after twenty-six years. Brooke has just moved into an apartment, and we gave him just about everything to get started.

Our visitors from Channel 13 stay for two hours and tape about twenty minutes of interviews, which are edited down to about ninety seconds. We become friends with Tina, who is a warm, compassionate, interesting lady. Brooke and Leah are sitting in the background watching. When it's over, Robert takes all of us to a late dinner at Logan's Roadhouse, which has just opened this week. I feel a rush of adrenaline after the interview, but Robert doesn't think he did well.

I have been weighing options for reconstructive surgery. My first choice is to have expanders inserted so my breasts can be increased in size over two or three months as the skin grows and adapts. But because of radiation, as I expected, this is not a viable approach. The skin on my right side just isn't elastic enough. So I must decide between a latissimus dorsi musculocutaneous flap or a transverse rectus abdominis musculocutaneous flap, called a TRAM. In the first case a block of skin and muscle from my back will be used to make a breast mound on each side. It provides a good blood supply, and an implant is usually needed. However, it leaves scars on my back—and I want very much to wear backless dresses. Robert thinks I have a pretty back, and I want to take advantage of whatever assets I have. The other choice, the TRAM, uses my stomach skin, fat, and muscle to create breasts. The result is soft, natural feeling breasts, and I have the added advantage of losing years of fat that has accumulated around my waist. I think long and hard about what to do, and I talk to several women who have had both procedures. I get mixed reviews, but the consensus is the TRAM. I really like the prospect of a tummy tuck as a bonus. Dr. Powell prepares me for at least six hours of surgery, three or four days hospitalization, and six weeks at home.

My feet have stopped itching, my hair is coming back again, and I detect the beginning of eyelashes and eyebrows. My heart palpitations are rare, and I feel wonderful. When I look into the mirror, I don't feel as freaky anymore. My face is starting to look like me again. Robert goes to a meeting in San Diego. Our builder, Rob, starts to clear our lot. I am busy getting my team ready for the Relay for Life. Robert and I have also gotten involved in a building campaign at church. Jessica goes to her senior prom. We are as busy as ever. But the surgery I will face on May 7 is utmost on my mind.

Two weeks before my TRAM flap, I must have a pedicle delay. This is a procedure where blood vessels in the lower abdomen are clipped to promote better blood flow to the tissue that will be transferred to my breast area. It is in essence surgery to get ready for surgery. On Wednesday, April 23, Robert delivers me to the Surgery Center. I'm escorted to Room 18 on the sixth floor. I get changed and become comfortable. Robert stays with me. My nurse is my friend, Robin. All my buddies from Outpatient Holding visit. Dr. Skilling comes in and gives me a warm hug. I feel calm and confident. I am enjoying the morning. Dr. Powell comes in and draws some marks on my tummy, and then it's time to go. Dr. Skilling intercepts us on the way and hands Robert another bunny suit to wear into the OR. My friend, George Myers, is the anesthetist. I see smiling faces everywhere. Robert and I agree that George smiles through his eyes. Robert holds my hand again. I hear lots of chitchat in the room, including a discussion about the camera. In what seems like a moment, I'm aware of my lower abdomen being mopped up, and I'm on the way to the Recovery Room. When I get home, I'm sore and take some pain medicine. I have learned not to rush into eating if there is any hint of nausea after anesthesia. I sleep well and realize the next day that I need to stay home until Monday. I was going to bounce back to work on Friday, but I don't feel like bouncing anywhere.

I am surprisingly sore and walk around like a hunched-over old lady. I have had a relatively minor procedure, which concerns me when I think about the real deal that is coming. I feel good enough to get out of the house, though, and Robert and I meet Rob at our lot to look at the way he has staked out the outline of the house. This is terribly exciting to finally walk around and say the kitchen is here, the garage is here, and this is the view from the patio. We found the house we wanted in Jacksonville and bought the plans from the builder. We haven't seen this floor plan anywhere in Macon, so we think we will have a unique home. Robert has ordered a custom-made address plate for the mailbox, and we take it out to show Rob for good luck.

The Relay for Life arrives. This is a packed weekend. Robert is speaking at the luminary ceremony Friday night, and then Brooke will be initiated into Robert's college fraternity on Saturday. Jessica goes with us to Northeast High School for the relay. We arrive about 4:00 P.M. well ahead of the deadline for setting up. The inside of the track is filling up with tents and all kinds of shelters. People are streaming in. This is an impressive sight. Everyone is enthusiastic. These people have been preparing for this event for months. Jessica volunteers at the Coca-Cola stand. We see Dr. Dale, who looks very official in his purple T-shirt. He's directing traffic and doing whatever needs to be done. I think it is great to see him out here and wish there were more doctors present to show their support. With so many doctors involved in some aspect of cancer treatment, their collective and individual response is disappointing to say the least.

Cancer survivors are supposed to put on a sash and a sticker that identify them, but I don't want to do this. I still don't want to wave my condition around like a banner and would prefer to look like just another volunteer. But my buddies and Robert keep urging me on, so I agree if my friend, Ken Bryant, will go with me. Ken has been through breast cancer during the same time period as I, and we have become very close. Ken says, "Let's go Rorie." So both of us report to the table where we get our sashes and sign a form where our names will be read during the survivor's walk.

At 6:00 P.M., it's time for the survivors to get their balloons and take a ceremonial lap around the track. I am thankful this is a walk and not a run. After several speeches, a large group of men and women of all ages walk around the track. This is a very moving and emotional few minutes. Halfway around, Robert decides to join me. I am glad to put my arms around him. He is a cancer survivor, too, in many ways. After the lap when the crowd starts to break up, Robert and I keep walking. A butterfly circles around us and will not leave. There are no other butterflies anywhere today that I've seen, but this one has landed on us and is determined to stay. I think my Daddy sent this symbol of new life to me, and he's telling me that I am emerging with a reborn spirit and body and maybe I'll be a symbol to someone else who needs strength. The little butterfly stays with us until we reach the spot where Daddy's candle is placed for the luminary ceremony, and then it gently flies away.

My buddies from the Medical Center keep arriving, and our friends from church are setting up an elaborate camp adjacent to us. We cook hamburgers and laugh and watch the sunset. At 10:00 P.M., a crowd gathers for the luminary ceremony in which thousands of candles are lit in honor of cancer survivors or in memory of those who were taken away by this awful disease. Robert is introduced. The crowd holds lighted candles while he speaks from his heart about why he's here. I am proud of him. He is able to capture the moment as the crowd listens in silence. When he comes down from the stage, we embrace, and friends surround us with hugs. We walk around the track and stop for a short prayer by Daddy's candle and then continue for several more laps as we watch this beautiful scene unfold. There is something almost holy about what is happening tonight. I feel connected to these people who are all here with very personal emotions.

On Saturday night, I attend a banquet for Brooke and his fraternity brothers honoring them for gaining a new charter. It is a black tie event, and all these young people look so handsome and optimistic. Brooke and Robert appear to be closer than I have ever seen them. At one point in the evening they embrace each other as father and son and as fraternity brothers. I cannot express how seeing them together like this fills my heart with joy.

It seems like a long time ago that we were interviewed in our living room, but tonight, the night before my surgery, we are on television. At about 4:45 P.M., Tina Hicks calls to remind us we will be the lead on the 5:00 o'clock early edition of the news. Robert and I gave our VCR to Brooke when he moved, but bought another one a couple of weeks ago, hoping to find a model that was idiot proof. The two of us have to experiment for about a half hour to figure out how to record. We wait anxiously for the program to start, Robert with remote control in hand, beaming with false confidence. We are both nervous because we have no idea what portions of the interview will be used and how the final product will be put together.

At the moment the program begins, the telephone rings. It is Hugh wishing me well. He offers a beautiful prayer as I see a photograph of Robert and me projected on the television screen. I am introduced as a woman who ignored symptoms and am now in for the fight of my life. The title of this series is "Friend for Life." The idea is that on the 13th day of each month a friend calls a friend to urge her to get a mammogram. Robert and I are pleased with how we are portrayed and see that Tina wants to treat us and our family with respect and affection while using me as an example of what not to do. Tina says that we have a beautiful family and a beautiful home, and at the end of the interview she remarks that it took a lot of courage for me to talk about my delaying tactics. I am very proud of her comments and begin to find it easier to express my feelings in public. I hope what I have said will help some woman who is stalling and afraid to get a mammogram.

Robert woke up Monday morning with unbearable pain in his right heel, but he hobbled to work. On Tuesday, he couldn't walk and stayed home. Now it is time to go to the hospital, and he is on crutches. When we arrive at 6:00 A.M. in the parking lot, Robert drags slowly behind me, and one wonders who is really the patient. As always, we are greeted with concern and care. We take the familiar elevator ride to the sixth floor and are assigned to Room 30. Like clockwork, Hugh arrives with his red hat and seems to enjoy sitting with us as he watches the sun rise over Macon. He gives us such comfort. When my nurse comes in, we all hold hands as Hugh offers a beautiful prayer and mentions faith, love, and peace beyond human understanding. Isn't that the truth? Everything that has happened to me is beyond human understanding. I don't know why I have done so well, but there is a reason, and I believe God is going to use me.

This is a good day, and good things are going to happen. Robert and I feel safe and secure. He's able to get some medication that helps the pain in his foot immediately. But he's very disappointed that he will not go into the OR with me. The crutches might be a safety hazard. I take some Valium and feel calm with a sense of wonderful anticipation. I wear my breast prostheses, but when I change into my hospital gown, I put them in my suitcase, never to wear them again.

Dr. Skilling comes in and hugs me. Soon Dr. Powell and Dr. Barron come in because it is time for me to be marked for surgery. I pull up my gown and stand all exposed with my flat, scarred chest for the last time. Dr. Powell draws lines on my stomach and chest as a guide to where the tissue will be transferred. He says he will use all the fat I have available around my tummy. This is the first time in my life I wish I had a little more to be moved up.

I'm on the way to the OR. It seems strange without Robert walking along beside the stretcher. I know he wants to be with me. My dear friend Brenda has a Yanni CD ready, and I am so thankful to have David and Dr. Skilling with me again. I am given a painless epidural. The next thing I know I am in the Recovery Room where I see Robert, Brooke, Jessica, and Leah. I am groggy but feel absolutely no pain. I am incredibly thirsty. Ice water has never tasted so good. After a short stay, it is time to be wheeled to Room 301, right down the hallway from the room where I stayed after my mastectomies.

I am in a scrunched-up position in bed to avoid any strain on my stomach, or at least what used to be my stomach. I peer down under my gown and see breast mounds and small steri-strips. Breast mounds! I haven't had breasts for eight months almost to the day. I have on a support bra that holds loose dressings around my new breasts. I also have a lightweight dressing on my new flat, trim stomach. I can't believe this is me. I have two drains from the stomach and one drain coming from each breast. I am used to drains from my previous surgery, but the last time, I lost my breasts. Now I have a new body, and I like it.

I have to be covered with a Bair Hugger, which we call a "bear hugger," a body heating device that increases blood circulation needed for healing. It is uncomfortably hot, and I need ice cold washcloths for my neck and the top of my head. Robert looks terrible. I insist he go home and get some rest. I can look out my window and see the building where I had my chemotherapy and wonder who might be in there right now finishing up a session. My nurse checks on me every hour during the first night to watch my circulation, temperature, color, and the amount of drainage. I can doze between checks, but I want to sleep more.

I see the sun rise for the second day in a row and believe it is God's way of greeting and urging me on. Hugh said something about the sunrise being a gift, and he is right as usual. I feel fine. The epidural is working because I have yet to have any pain. My friends come by, and I am receiving phone calls and flowers. I am not hungry, but I manage to take in some of my liquid diet that is provided. I have lots of equipment around me again. I have a Foley catheter, an epidural box, and IVs for antibiotics and fluids. Robert arrives and looks much better. He helps me with a sponge bath. It feels good to brush my teeth and put on some lipstick. I took off my wig yesterday before surgery and have left it off. My friends have seen the real me. My extremely short new hair is almost fashionable.

Dr. Dale, Dr. Skilling, and Dr. Barron come by. David checks on me and gives me a hug. When Dr. Powell comes in, he says he is extremely pleased, and I have done as well as any patient he has ever had. He shows Robert my new breasts. It is difficult to believe how natural they look. Dr. Powell has again lived up to his reputation as an artist. This is wonderful. This is really wonderful. He tells me he is glad I feel so well, but not to be surprised if I have a bad day. It is common to have a swing in the recovery pattern from day to day.

Dr. Powell was right. It is Friday, and I am having some waves of nausea. I think it may be the Fentanyl in my epidural that makes me feel bad, so I have it removed and start to improve right away. I have oral pain medication on hand, but I don't need it. This afternoon I am free of all the tubes except the drains. My catheter is gone, the epidural is history, and my IVs are unplugged. I am able to get myself into the bathroom and can almost straighten up, though I am still extremely tight around the middle.

Kelly Crissman from church visits me, and we have a stimulating talk. This is the first time I have really had a conversation with Kelly since he became our associate pastor. I love the way he listens and finds such meaning in what goes on around us. He tells me that Hugh has gone up to northwest Georgia for two days in the mountains. I am glad because he looked tired and burdened with our building campaign when he came to see me on Wednesday. Hugh mentioned that the mountains give him strength and that's just where he needed to go. Late today Robert leaves to pick up a flower dish for Mother's Day. There is a powerful storm, and one of our firemen is killed by a fallen tree. This is such a tragedy. Robert gets caught in the storm on the interstate and tells me it was unbelievable. Tonight, Jessica is mistress of ceremonies at a church production to raise money for the youth to take a mission trip to Costa Rica. I wish I could be in the Fellowship

Hall watching the show, a murder mystery in which Jessica is the victim. Robert and Brooke attend and report that it is an entertaining evening.

I don't sleep well and end up watching an old Mary Tyler Moore rerun at 4:30 A.M. I am mobile, so I putter around my room and give myself a sponge bath and put on some makeup. No one seems appalled to see my very short hair, so I'll forget the wig for a while. It is so much cooler with it off. I see the sun rise for the third day and thank God for His greeting. Robert comes by early and brings me a McDonald's muffin and the newspaper and then goes home to do some long overdue yardwork. Dr. Powell tells me I will be able to go home tomorrow, which is Mother's Day. That will be my gift.

Brooke arrives, and then Hugh comes in with his red hat and a container of oil for anointing. We have a short but exhilarating ceremony with a prayer while Hugh anoints my head with oil. Here I am with Hugh and Brooke, and my spirit soars. I still have not needed any pain medication. I know that my spirit must be keeping the pain away. Every doctor and nurse who comes in the room tells me how people are talking about me and how well I am doing. It is almost embarrassing, but again I know God is using me, and God has a plan.

Robert arrives early and looks so good. I am ready to go home. I have seen the sun rise again. This Mother's Day is beautiful beyond description. I have received the best of care and have made new friends with a great team of nurses. I eat a big breakfast of eggs, bacon, grits, biscuits, coffee, and orange juice. I can stand straight up and walk with ease. I get dressed and hide my drains in my stretch pants and put my blonde wig on. My wig is my security blanket; I'm not quite ready for the world to see my head. I'm given pain medication to take home, but I don't think I'll need it. It's time to go. Robert leaves to get the Jeep so he can pick me up at Patient Dismissal. When we pull away from the Medical Center, I have one of my little cries because I am so happy and blessed with God's grace. My long journey is almost over, and God has delivered me safely home.

I am anxious to resume my normal household activities, but I know I have to take it easy, even though I am not experiencing any pain. Just going up the stairs tires me out. I need to nap frequently, and I feel a bit lightheaded. Robert is trying to help any way he can.

He washes the sheets and mops the kitchen floor. I refuse to whine, but I do need help—and I get all I need.

I can see the ridges of muscle that were stretched up to my chest. They cross over my diaphragm forming a bulge. The muscles are sort of flexed right now, but some of the nerves were cut, so they will relax eventually, and the bulge between my new breasts will disappear. My new breasts look wonderful. They are soft, pink, and warm. The circulation is as good as can possibly be expected. My belly button was moved up when my stomach was stitched back together, and I got another innie. My stomach is so flat, it's almost concave. It looks as though I have devoted years to sit-ups. I feel like I have cheated, but I'll take it. Boy, will I take it! The incision on my stomach is very tidy and forms a big smile that will be hidden by a bathing suit. I think I may actually be able to venture back to a bikini, but I will have to wait a few months to see. All that remains is the addition of nipples. I most certainly will want to get some implants to increase the breast size a bit. Both of those procedures may happen at the same time and can be done on an outpatient basis. After what I've been through, that little bit of surgery will be a piece of cake. I will have to wait about ten weeks for everything to heal nicely, and then Dr. Powell will complete his artwork.

My first night home, sleep comes easily in my own bed with Robert next to me. My emotions can only be described as uncontrollable joy. Robert stays home with me on Monday. I get calls and cards, and Brenda, my dear angel of a friend, shows up with chicken parmesan, risotto, carrot cake, and a bottle of wine. She hasn't seen our new pooch, Peanut, but she picks her up and says, "What a little peanut!" We must have picked the right name to fit the personality.

Brooke and Leah have broken up, and experience tells me that a parent needs to stay out of a grown child's affairs. But it saddens me to see them drift apart. Leah is just like my daughter, and I would be happy if they got married. She has been a part of our family for several years, and I have grown to love her. I know that what will be will be, but it is not easy for me to keep from intervening. I pray for the best for both of them.

Robert goes to work late on Tuesday because he wants to stay with me, but he also has an important meeting he can't miss. He returns home early, and we go see Dr. Powell together. My drains will have to stay in for a few more days at least, and I'm told to continue to measure the volume of fluids and call on Friday morning. I would like to have these things removed before the weekend, but I understand how important it is to rid myself of the bodily fluids resulting from my surgery. Robert gets the first total look at my stomach and breasts, and he seems to accept their appearance. When I recover, I will have nicely-shaped breasts. In some ways they may be better, but I will always have scars—though they will fade over time.

On Wednesday, I continue to feel better, but I am tired. I am convinced that prayer and attitude really do reduce pain because I have yet to take any medicine. This afternoon the drain coming from my left breast falls out. Since so little fluid is evident, I just put some gauze over the opening and keep it clean. I sit outside to feel the warmth of the sun and start to work on a tan from lotion out of a bottle. When Robert gets home, we ride out to look at the house construction and are thrilled to see that most of the concrete block foundation is complete.

Robert and I have always loved each other, but we have also remained in love. There is a difference. I know so many married couples who truly love each other, but as time passes I wonder if they are still *in* love. I'm referring to the kind of passion couples have during the early part of their marriage. I have recalled so many times why I fell in love with Robert. I enjoy his humor, his sensitivity, and his talent. He has always been able to make me laugh. But the most important thing has always been the hundreds of ways he shows his love for me.

This has been the most difficult year of my life and of his. I think one reason couples who love each other may not continue to be in love is because we think after a certain number of years, there is nothing left to be discovered. One of the miracles of my encounter with breast cancer is that Robert and I have discovered feelings about each other and beliefs in God that we might have never otherwise disclosed. A situation that could have destroyed us has resulted in a stronger love and deeper understanding.

We have walked through the fire together hand in hand, protected by an army of angels. And we know each one of those angels because they have the names and faces of friends and family we love. Those angels have prayed for us and kept us in their thoughts every day. They have sent beautiful cards and letters and brought food and gifts I will always cherish. They have called us and cheered us on. And they have understood the wigs and the times when I was tired and not feeling like myself. Those angels have always been nearby creating a healing bridge between God and my body and soul. As Robert and I come to the end of this miraculous chapter in our lives, we will never forget their love. My faith tells me that God will continue to make His plan more apparent to me. I will never forget what has happened. I am ready to follow God's will wherever it may lead me.

From Robert . . .

It is difficult to stand up in front of the congregation and talk from my heart about cancer and what it has done to my family over the past year. I am standing in the same spot where Tim Bagwell stood when he had to tell our church about Susan. I know that the feelings I have are much the same as Tim had on that painful Sunday. By a stroke of luck, I suppose, Rorie's surgery is on the Wednesday after the Relay for Life, and the day after our interview by Tina Hicks at Channel 13 will be broadcast.

I think a great deal about the Relay for Life and feel honored to be asked to speak at the beginning of the luminary ceremony. In fact, I believe I was recommended by Tim. I want to say something appropriate and meaningful and am determined not to let my emotions detract from the message. As I approach the microphone, I feel a sense of calmness—as though I am supposed to be here. Night has fallen. I cannot see the faces in the crowd, only handheld candle after candle. A peacefulness permeates the scene that helps me talk intimately with those who have decided to participate in the ceremony. I say,

> *I have been a part of three Relays for Life. The first two years I came because it was the right thing to do. I am here tonight because it is the only thing to do. I have to be here. Why are you here? I think you're here because you love someone. I'm here because I love my wife who has been fighting breast cancer since last year. And I'm here because I love my father-in-law who lost*

his life to multiple myeloma. And I'm here because I have good friends with a little girl who has leukemia. And I'm here because I know many of you who are fighting cancer in your life. I think you're here because you love someone who has lost the fight with cancer. And I think you're here because you love someone who has won the fight with cancer. And I think you're here because you love someone who you want to never face this dreadful disease.

We become experts because we want to or because we have to. All of us have become experts because we have to. We will laugh and cry and walk because we must do whatever must be done. We will be here next year and the year after and the year after until we don't have to fight anymore. What we have done already will make a difference as we help our doctors and researchers save more lives.

When I was a little boy, I couldn't tell if Jesus said I am the Light or if Jesus said I am the Life. But after thinking about it, it didn't matter because Jesus could have said both. We cannot have life without light. Jesus is our Light, and Jesus is our Life. So every light tonight symbolizes the life of someone we love. Go now and find the light of the life that you love.

I am glad that Hugh and Becky are close by listening. They hug me when I step down from the stage, and Hugh tells me he's proud of me. That means more to me than he realizes. Rorie and Jessica and I walk several laps and then load up the Jeep and drive away slowly. The view from the hill overlooking the track is almost heavenly as the darkness is broken by thousands of candles including the word "Hope" rising up the gentle slope for everyone to see.

I am disappointed on Saturday because I cannot return, but this day will be Brooke's day, and I must share it with him. Brooke graduated from Mercer University more than a year ago but was not able to be initiated into his fraternity because at the time it had not regained its charter. But today is the day my son will be initiated into Sigma Alpha Epsilon as I was twenty-nine years ago. I meet Brooke at the fraternity house for lunch with the impressive young men who will be initiated. Then all of us take a short ride to a local church where the ceremony will take place.

The initiation will be conducted by several officials from the national fraternity office and the fraternity province. It is discovered that they are one man short for the initiation team, and I am offered the job—which I enthusiastically accept. Not only will I be able to pin Brooke; I will help officiate throughout the entire ceremony. I find to my great delight and astonishment that the official directing the ceremony is the same man who conducted my initiation in Tampa on January 20, 1968. He tells me he remembers me. Though it is doubtful, I want to believe him—so I do. We initiate forty-six wonderful young men. When we step in front of Brooke, I say, "This is my son," and place his fraternity pin on his shirt. We are now father and son, brother and brother. This is one of the proudest moments of my life. I say a silent prayer thanking God for this very good day after so many that have been painful.

The festivities carry on into the evening when a banquet is held to recognize the new brothers and to present awards. Wives and dates are included. Rorie and Leah enjoy themselves. The national president of the fraternity remarks that the room is full of the most beautiful women, not only in the South, but in the world. The young ladies escorted by these newly initiated fraternity men are indeed beautiful. On the way home, it is excruciatingly evident how Rorie's struggle has become such an integral part of my consciousness. I turn to her and observe that of the forty-six or so beautiful young women present at the dinner, at least five will one day be diagnosed with breast cancer. I pray some new breakthrough treatment proves me wrong.

We are thrilled with the way Channel 13 presents our story on television. Rorie is magnificent as she uses her courage and faith to tell everyone that she was full of denial and waited too long to go to the doctor. She is willing to open up one of the most intimate truths in her personal life in order to warn other women and assure them that God and a concerned doctor can get them through this frightful experience. We later learn that the station receives 170 calls on Tuesday night after our segment. Something Rorie said must have touched many, many people.

On Wednesday morning I can only walk with crutches. This is the most severe pain I have ever experienced. I can't imagine why my right heel hurts as it does. The only cause I can think of is an attack of gout. I would do anything to stay home in bed nursing my swollen foot, but I cannot miss this day of all days. As Rorie and I enter the Surgery Center, I am prepared for the questions and jokes about me being the one who needs to be hospitalized. Rorie is excited and full of her trademark confidence. Her only concern seems to be for me.

Jessica arrives a few minutes after we check into the room, with Brooke and Hugh following close behind. I hop and skip around the room, going from the chair to Rorie's bed. Brooke is highly entertained. Rorie changes into her hospital gown, takes off her wig, and then puts on some special stockings to prevent blood clots during surgery. I'm amused that these stockings have holes in the bottom so they can be pushed back to take a pulse in the foot. The thought of more holes in our socks comes to mind. Hugh stays with us, and we talk about the sunrise, mountains, and the story behind his red hat.

Jessica, Brooke, and Hugh have to leave. Soon Roy Powell and Tim Barron come in to get Rorie marked for surgery. Roy looks like a sculptor drawing on a piece of marble that will become a work of art. I look at Rorie's mastectomy-scarred chest for the last time and try to envision what the results of reconstruction will look like. At 8:35 A.M., the stretcher is brought in. I feel frustrated that my crutches prevent me from going into the OR. I kiss Rorie and tell her I love her. Suddenly, I am all alone.

I say a prayer and thank God for this incredible day and for bringing Rorie and me to this destination. I sit quietly and marvel at the beautiful day we have to celebrate, and then I close my eyes for a while and try to forget about the pain in my foot. This is a day for joy, and I don't want to be hobbling around answering questions about why I'm limping.

Brenda calls from the OR at 9:15 and tells me Rorie is asleep and surgery is starting. She calls again at 10:25 and at 11:20 with reports that everything is going extremely well. At 12:10 P.M., she calls and tells me Roy is creating a new bellybutton. Then, at 1:20, Brenda calls to say Rorie's tummy is all gone and Roy is beginning to stitch up her new breasts. All of this seems incredible. Surgery will be over in about forty-five minutes to an hour. Hugh returns at 1:35 and wants me to call him at church as soon as Rorie is in recovery. He will give a report at the Wednesday night supper.

In between calls from Brenda, Leah has arrived and stays most of the morning. Melinda and Terri from my office bring the day's paperwork that needs my signature. Terri's husband, Dr. Bill Terry, calls in a prescription for an anti-inflammatory drug. Brooke and Leah bring me lunch from the cafeteria and also my prescription, which works right away.

Brenda calls at 2:30. The surgery is a grand success, and Rorie soon will be in the Recovery Room. I should go to Outpatient Holding and find an empty room to meet with Roy. It's over. It's finally over. Thank you, God, and thank you, Dr. Powell.

Brooke, Leah, and I go directly to Outpatient Holding. In about five minutes Roy comes in and tells us the surgery went about as well as any he has ever performed. He tells me the right side is still very tight, and the left breast may end up slightly larger, but nothing can be determined until the swelling goes down and gravity takes over. A small implant may be indicated on the right or maybe implants on both sides. Roy smiles at me when he says Rorie will probably opt for implants on both sides, and I say it's a sure thing. I wait outside the Recovery Room propped up on my crutches. I have to tell everyone who walks by why I can't walk. I use the gout story because it works, so I decide to stick to it. After about fifteen minutes, I can finally go in to see Rorie.

Her color is kind of gray at first, and she is very groggy. But in a few minutes after drinking some ice water, her color is good, and she is fully awake and reports no pain. She has on some sort of heating device that will keep her circulation up and help with healing. With all the covering, I cannot detect any results of the surgery, but Rorie's beaming face and smile convince me it is a success. I call her mother from the Recovery Room, and she picks up the phone with one ring. Mary's voice is full of relief when I tell her Rorie is awake and doing well. As a former Army nurse, Mary has been extremely worried about Rorie being under anesthesia for so many hours. As any mother would be, she has been on pins and needles all day waiting for my call. The kids come in, and then we're off to Room 301.

Rorie's room has to be kept very warm, so the thermostat is set on 85 degrees. It feels hotter. She is flushed, and her face is puffy. I put a washcloth in some ice and place it on her head—which she loves. We have become accustomed to excellent nurses, and her care is once again superb. I am so proud of Rorie who has people all around the Medical Center talking about how well she has done. This day is full of blessings, but I cannot ignore the fact that I feel awful. My foot is much better, but the medication is making me pay a price with a stomach ache. I reluctantly go home and do not spend the night in Rorie's room. But the rest I get is God-sent.

On Thursday, we have a happy day. Father Bob comes by, and we hold hands and pray. He offers the most moving and powerful prayers that affect the healing process. We are blessed to have him as a friend and chaplain. Reverend Tim Price is at a conference out of town. We know he is praying for us, too. Rorie and I are grateful when Kelly Crissman visits. We enjoy listening to him and are struck by how observant he is. Rorie gives him a thumbs up when he asks how she feels, and he tells us how his little boy always wants Daddy to do the same. Kelly is having a difficult day and tells Rorie how she is ministering to him. How remarkable that is, I think, that Rorie's words and attitude are providing comfort to our associate minister. Kelly sees clearly how there are connections in this life, and I see a lasting friendship connecting between him and Rorie.

The room is filling with flowers and cards and other presents, but the one that produces the most laughter and interest is Fireman Fred. It's a date-in-the-box and includes a photograph of a handsome young fireman and some so-called personal notes and cards. Rorie's fireman thing must be legendary. I hear later that one of her nurse friends has actually cornered a fireman in the hallway and is trying to convince him to come to Rorie's room for a visit. I ask Rorie exactly what will she do if the fireman comes in. I get a smile but no definitive answer. I guess the firemen who come into the Medical Center have no idea what they're up against.

Rorie progresses and is standing up straight by Saturday. I leave early to do some housecleaning and to run some errands. I want to arrive early Sunday to bring Rorie home. The wig has gone back on but not for long. This is Mother's Day. It is one of the most beautiful days we have seen in weeks. Before we get home, we ride by our lot. There are stacks of concrete blocks ready for the workers to start on the foundation. Rorie says how grateful she is that her body has been rebuilt, so now she can start thinking about building our house. We get unpacked, and Rorie stretches out in the living room. We are amazed when the afternoon movie turns out to be none other than *Fried Green Tomatoes*. There's the Whistle Stop Cafe. We make plans to have lunch there again as soon as Rorie is able.

Brenda brings us a fabulous Italian dinner, and I think how she is not only a nurse angel but a gourmet chef angel. She is such a friend to us. I am very touched by all the gestures of love she provides. Rorie and I sit at the kitchen table eating this delicious meal and talk about all that has happened to us over the past year. I remark that as painful as it has been, I feel as though we have been carried through with God's spirit holding us up. We will never know how many people have prayed nor how many prayers have been offered on our behalf. But we know that intercessory prayer by many people who love us has brought us to this point where we have most certainly won our battle.

The church bulletin will arrive on Friday. I have requested that it be the last time Rorie's name appears in the Circle of Concern. It will mark forty-eight consecutive weeks her name has appeared, and this Sunday will conclude forty-nine consecutive Sabbaths when Rorie's name has been lifted up in church asking for healing. Our friends and family have cared for us and loved us, and God has listened. I will never be the same human being I was a year ago. God has taken me and shaken my spirit so that I will be a better husband, father, brother, and friend. He has challenged me to love more deeply, hope more confidently, and live more sincerely.

It is absolutely essential for Rorie and me to get some closure on this year of our greatest heartbreaks and our greatest joys. We've been knocked down, but we've been lifted up, and our love and understanding for each other have increased a thousandfold. Last June, we were two frightened people who were terrified of a mammogram report waiting for us when we returned from a short trip to Panama City Beach. Now we are going to the beach again and will sit in the exact spot one year to the day where we watched that beautiful sunset as our fears overwhelmed us. This time, our hearts will be full of the joy God has given us. Rorie's hair will be different, her body will not be the same, and we'll both be a year older. But we'll bury our feet in the sand and hold on to each other just like two lovers on their honeymoon. And do you know what? We won't be the least surprised if that angel reappears and helps us capture that special moment beginning our new life together on Somersby Lane.

CANCER AS TEACHER
Lessons Learned

"I pray that you will begin to understand how incredibly great His power is to help those who believe Him."

—Ephesians 1:19 LB

Breast cancer is a relentless and ruthless teacher that has no compassion for its pupils. It demands complete attention and cruelly presses onward with a vengeance toward destroying the body and the soul. It shows no favoritism and desperately wants each member of the class to fail. But with all its power to rip away the fabric of life, it is no match for faith, hope, and love.

We have learned from breast cancer. The lessons we were exposed to on a daily basis are common to many who have suffered from this frightening disease, and perhaps a few are unique to our experience. Regardless, we pray that those with breast cancer, and also those who love someone with this disease will be able to learn something helpful from our newfound convictions.

Lesson 1: *As the greatest physician, God appreciates the value of a referral.* God has given our doctors an arsenal of treatments and the will to find a cure. We began our story describing many months of denial and postponement that allowed the cancer to advance to a Stage III carcinoma. This was totally preventable. Our prayer above all else is that every woman will perform regular breast self-examinations and get a mammogram. Husbands and wives need to overcome their fears and seek medical care at the first hint of a lump in the breast. We are experts at denial, and we understand the overwhelming power of fear. God wants us to have faith, but at the same time God wants us to seek out earthly assistance. We need prayer, but we also need a good doctor.

Lesson 2: *Make sure your doctor understands that hope is a vital part of the practice of medicine.* This lesson is closely related to the first. We have heard repeatedly from our doctors that attitude and faith had an enormous effect on the healing process. The lack of pain medication Rorie needed after reconstructive surgery was a clear example of the power of positive emotions. As medical advances become more effective, some physicians act as though their technical skill is all that is necessary. They forget that for most of the history of medicine, physicians could do little but stay at the bedside and hold the patient's hand and offer hope and comfort. That aspect of the practice of medicine is just as important today. Unfortunately, we regularly observe a small number of medical students, residents, and practicing physicians who get into the most human of professions without having any detectable people skills. Some seem not to have acquired even the most basic communication skills such as the ability to smile and say "Good morning" in the hallway.

Even physicians who base their entire approach to healing on science alone can no longer ignore the evidence. In a California study on the effect of prayer on recovery from heart problems, half of nearly 400 patients were the subjects of prayer. Neither of the two groups studied were told about the intercessory prayer that was occurring. The group that was the focus of prayer had half as many complications. A Dartmouth Medical School study tracked how patients' own prayers helped them to recover from bypass surgery. Those who prayed regularly had a lower death rate. Harvard has hosted a conference for doctors on Spirituality and Healing in Medicine. An American Academy of Family Physicians survey showed that 99% of physicians believe there is an important relationship between the body and the spirit. One wonders why more physicians aren't prescribing prayer. It is at least as effectve as some of our medications.

Lesson 3: *Cancer is not an infectious disease.* We will forever be grateful for the overwhelming love and attention we received from friends all over the country. We heard from friends we have not talked with in years, and some of our angels sent as many as four or five cards over the course of this most difficult year. But we are saddened that several of our personal and professional friends never once responded to our most basic need to know they cared. The silence has been deafening. We have seen too many examples of people who apparently cope best by avoiding the reality of what is happening. We certainly understand the seductive value of denial. Please, if friends are going through a life-threatening crisis, let them know you care. For a long time, we wouldn't even say the word "cancer"—evidently some of us think it is infectious. We all want to avoid what is unpleasant, but we hope this experience has taught us to be more responsive to friends who need a kind word and a demonstration of concern.

Lesson 4: *Avoid doomsdayers.* Just as it is vitally important to hear encouragement from friends and family, it is equally important to avoid those who deliver gloom and doom. There is no shortage of people who will fill your time with stories of how they or someone they know became violently sick from chemotherapy. One nurse administrator at the hospital, who never once inquired as to how we were doing, did on one occasion go out of her way to describe how rough treatment would be. While we have always appreciated and welcomed questions about how we are doing, some individuals seem capable of only an interrogation about the quality of care and the wisdom of a particular choice of therapy. Seek out people who radiate a positive glow, and run to the hills from those who drain your energy and confidence.

Lesson 5: *The way you look affects the way you feel.* It is terribly painful to lose one's hair. But if it is going to happen, get a short haircut right away. It lessens the trauma as the hair comes out. Wigs can be an opportunity to become the blonde or redhead you always thought about. Salon wigs are often the most expensive, and there is very little relationship between price and what looks good on you. The least expensive wigs from a catalog can be the most flattering and realistic. Take special care to wear clothes that make you feel attractive. Pay extra attention to grooming and makeup. And remember that humor is one of God's greatest gifts. Look for humor, and find opportunities for laughter. Nothing can make you feel and look better than a smile.

Lesson 6: *Breast cancer is not the end of a sexual relationship.* It is not easy to talk about one of the most personal aspects of life. A mastectomy can signal a decrease in sexual activity due to fear or a reduction in desire on the part of one or both partners. While the period following a mastectomy requires untold patience and understanding, normal sexual relations can and should continue. The closeness and bond between husband and wife during this time are critically important to maintain. Some reconstructive techniques can be performed immediately after mastectomy, thus avoiding any loss of the presence of a breast mound. If there is delay in reconstruction, partners can continue to be intimate with the assurance that the absence of one or both breasts is only temporary.

Lesson 7: *Listen more, look more, and love more.* Breast cancer changes everything. But it doesn't have to change everything for the worse. Even in this terrible situation, there is opportunity. It is important to slow down and reevaluate what and who are really important in life. It is a gift in a way because we listened to each other more closely than ever, and we became more sensitive to people and events around us. So many aspects of life that we had taken for granted gained significance. The love between us as husband and wife grew stronger, and the love for family and friends grew deeper. One of the greatest miracles is that we were able to grow close to many people who might otherwise have been acquaintances only. Breast cancer has brought wonderful people into our lives who have blessed us with their strength, love, and special kindness.

Lesson 8: *Turn to God, and go to church.* We have saved the most important lesson for last. Psalm 46 tells us that God is our refuge and strength, an everpresent help in trouble. When we found ourselves in trouble, God's church came to our rescue. God sent love to us through our ministers and church friends who continue to call and pray and lift our spirits. We were able to hear God's message on Sunday mornings through Hugh Davis' powerful sermons and the angels singing in the choir. The prayerful cards and letters we received from Tim and Susan Bagwell are among our earthly treasures. During the darkest hours, God would speak to us in the quietest moments. We are no longer afraid. We look to God to reveal His plan to us for the rest of our lives. On the day before we completed this book, our labor of love, we received a card from a dear friend, Jimmie Powell. The inscription was from Jeremiah 29:11 (NIV), and it beautifully captures the dream we hold in our hearts.

> *"For I know the plans I have for you, declares the Lord, plans to prosper you and not to harm you, plans to give you hope and a future."*

AFTERWORD

Upon learning that my wife had struggled with breast cancer, a misinformed but well-meaning person stated, "So you are a breast cancer victim." Patiently, but with an edge in her voice, my wife corrected the statement: "No, I am a breast cancer survivor." Such is the spirit displayed in the pages you have read.

Breast cancer is insidious, striking fear into the hearts of those who face it. As one who is married to a woman who has faced breast cancer on two occasions, I am keenly aware of the ravages of the disease, not only on the patient but also on all those close to her.

There are some who respond to the trauma by becoming victims of their situation. Emotionally and spiritually, their world crumbles. Fear controls all relationships important to them. Sometimes fear causes women to deny what is happening, not wanting to share in the process of decision making.

There are others who face breast cancer as genuine survivors. Defining survival simply in physiological terms is far too narrow. As a pastor, I have watched some women with very poor prognoses move through a face-to-face encounter with death. They died with dignity. Surviving has much more to do with spirit. Some of my friends who have died of breast cancer or other manifestations of cancer are as much survivors as those who live with the disease. There is a certain spirit that captures the proper definition of survival.

It is this spirit of survival that Robert and Rorie Fore have portrayed so well in their story. They understand that surviving does not mean denying the reality of the trauma and fear. As you have witnessed their struggle, you have seen normal, natural, and healthy tears. However, you also have had the opportunity to laugh and applaud as you have read the intimate account of how this couple faced the disease together. In the tears, laughter, smiles, and even the moments of silence one word leaps out as describing their response to breast cancer. That word is survival.

Without a doubt, this book is ministry. The practical advice offered concerning medical issues is invaluable. The vulnerable way in which Robert and Rorie share their emotions gives strength to those who face similar circumstances. But most important, their understanding of suffering within the context of faith is deeply moving. Instead of going it on their own, the Fores relied on their friends, family, church, and pastors to keep them focused on the healing power of God. Their very lives reflect an affirmation of faith.

Victims or survivors? Whatever the clinical prognosis might be, the Fores have provided the reader with a glimpse of a path that leads in the direction of survival. What a hopeful, godly way of living! So while this story is about a couple facing the daily struggles that come with breast cancer, its true theme is more encompassing. It deals, too, with the human condition and how we are to live our lives in the face of suffering.

—Timothy J. Bagwell